The Development *of* Medicine *for* OCR GCSE

Lomas

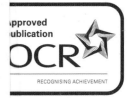
Approved
Publication
OCR
RECOGNISING ACHIEVEMENT

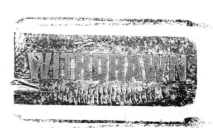

This book is for Fran, Ryland, Becky, Matty and Joe.

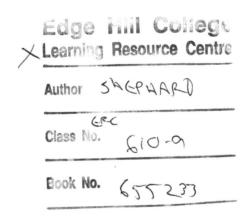
Orders: please contact Bookpoint Ltd, 130 Milton Park, Abingdon, Oxon OX14 4SB.
Telephone: (44) 01235 827720. Fax: (44) 01235 400454. Lines are open from 9.00 -
6.00, Monday to Saturday, with a 24 hour message answering service. You can also
order through our website www.hodderheadline.co.uk

British Library Cataloguing in Publication Data
A catalogue record for this title is available from the British Library

ISBN 0 340 78976X

First Published 2003
Impression number   10 9 8 7 6 5 4 3 2 1
Year   2009 2008 2007 2006 2005 2004 2003

Copyright © 2003 Colin Shephard

Typeset by Endangered Species, Essex.
Printed in Italy for Hodder & Stoughton Educational, a division of Hodder Headline,
338 Euston Road, London NW1 3BH.

Contents

Acknowledgements

The front cover illustration shows The Triumph of Death MSS 1503, Death of Laura due to the Black Death 1348, Poetry of Petrarch, 1304-1374, AA334460; reproduced courtesy of The Art Archive/Bibliothèque Nationale, Paris/Joffe.

The publishers would like to thank the following individuals, institutions and companies for permission to reproduce copyright illustrations in this book: © AKG London, pages 8, 76, 82 (top right); AKG London/Erich Lessing, page 65; AP Photo/Benny Gool, page 163; © Archivo Iconografico, S.A./Corbis, page 116; © The Art Archive, pages 43, 80, 111 (right), 154; © Bettman/Corbis, pages 91 (left), 91 (bottom right), 98, 113 (top), 119, 153; Bibliothèque Nationale, Paris LAT 6966 fol 4 RCC 2430, page 69; Christ healing a leper in the Echternach Gospels Lectionary (mid-11th century) ms 9428, fol. 23, recto, Bibliothèque Royale Albert 1er, Brussels, page 57 (bottom); Bodleian Library MS Rawlings B124f 197v Oxford, page 68 (top); Lion and Porcupine by Villard de Honnecourt, Bibliothèque Nationale, Paris/The Bridgeman Art Library, London, page 90 (top); Roy 16 F II f. 73 Tower of London and shipping, with Charles, Duke of Orleans seated in the Tower writing, c.1500, British Library, London/Bridgeman Art Library, page 79; Credit: Sketch of a ward at the hospital at Scutari, c.1856, Joseph-Austin Benwell, 19[th]c. English/Greater London Council, UK/The Bridgeman Art Library, London, page 156 (top); Living Made Easy: Prescription for Scolding Wives, printed by J. Netherclift, pub. 1830 by T. McLean (print), Private collection/The Bridgeman Art Library, London, 147; English School (18th c.) Leg Amputation (Panel), Royal College of Surgeons, London, UK/Bridgeman Art Library, London, page 142; MS CCC 123 f.29 Zodiac Man, from a calendar or astrological notes, English 14th–15th century (parchment), Corpus Christi College, Oxford, UK/Bridgeman Art Library, page 68 (bottom); © The British Library Cotton Aug AV1 fol 66, page 71; © The British Library MS 2572, fol 50 recto, page 73 (right); © The British Library MS Sloane 1977 fol 50.v., page 73 (left); © The British Library Sloan 1977 fol 50v, page 74; © The British Library Roy 15 DI 18, page 75; © The British Library Add. MS 19720 f. 27 Building a country house by Petrus de Crescentiis, 15th Century French Manuscript, page 78; © The British Library C.54.k.12 fol. Tp, page 93 (bottom); © The British Museum, pages 22, 30, 47, 54; Carlsberg Glypotek Museum, Copenhagen, page 18 (left); CDC/Science Photo Library, page 164; A History of Technology, Vol II (The Clarendon Press, 1956), page 77; © Corbis, page 145 (right); © Deutsches Archäologisches Institut-Athen, pages 26, 27, 33, 34; C.M. Dixon, Canterbury, page 49; © The Egypt Exploration Society, 3 Doughty Mews, London WC1N 2PG, page 18 (right); Mary Evans Picture Library, page 97; Gustave Doré in London, a Pilgrimage/Mary Evans, page 124; Amedee Forestier in the Illustrated London News, 9/1/09, p53/Mary Evans, page 139; © The Fotomas Index, UK, page 100 (all); Foto Roncaglia, page 85; © Guildhall Library, Corporation of London, page 130 (bottom left); Index, Florence/Ravenna, page 66; © Hulton Archive, page 100; © Hulton-Deutsch Collection/Corbis, pages 122, 132, 136, 138, 149 (top); © Hulton Getty, pages 104 (top), 115; EH Shepard, Punch, Centre for the Study of Cartoons and Caricature, University of Kent, Canterbury, page 141 (top); Zec from the Daily Mirror, 1945 © J. Churchill, The Mirror (Strips and Cartoons), Centre for the Study of Cartoons and Caricature, University of Kent, Canterbury, page 141 (bottom); Kunsthistorisches Museum mit MUK und ÖTM, Vienna, page 86 (centre); © Emma Lee/Life File, page 45; Mitchell Library, page 128; Hank Morgan/Science Photo Library, page 165; Musée Départemental d'art ancien et contemporain à Épinal–Vosges Photo by Christian Voegtlé, page 38; Museum of London, page 58; © Michael Nicholson/Corbis, page 91 (top); By courtesy of the National Portrait Gallery, London, page 156 (bottom); Photo RMN – H. Lewandowski, page 25; Photothèque du Musée de l'homme, page 9 (top and left); © The Pierpont Morgan Library/Art Resource, NY, page 67; Popperfoto, page 15; Punch, pages 125, 129, 133, 160; The Royal Collection © HM Queen Elizabeth II, page 90 (bottom); Scala/Chiesa dei Quattro, page 57 (top); Scala/Museo Nazionale Atestino, page 50; Science Museum, page 126 (left); Science & Society Picture Library, Science Museum, page 10; Ronald Sheridan/Ancient Art and Architecture Collection, page 52; Constellations of the Zodiac: Sagittarius and Capricornicus. Folio from a 'Aja-ib al-Makhluqat by Muhammad al-Qazwin, Freer Gallery of Art, Smithsonian Institution, Washington, D.C.: Purchase, 1954.45r Iraq 1350/1400, page 86 (top); Stonyhurst College, page 82 (bottom right); Wellcome Library, London, pages 20, 40, 42, 72, 82 (bottom left), 93 (top), 95, 107, 108, 109, 111 (left), 113 (centre), 130 (top left), 130 (right), 134 (left), 135, 145 (left), 146, 148, 151; Wellcome Photo Library, pages 104 (bottom), 155, 158.

The publishers would also like to thank the following for permission to reproduce material in this book: Professor M.L. Cameron for extracts and extracts that have been adapted from Anglo-Saxon Medicine by M.L. Cameron (Cambridge University Press, 1993); Constable & Robinson for the extract from Source Book of Medical History by Logan Clendening (Constable & Co, 1942); HarperCollins Publishers for the extracts from The Greatest Benefit to Mankind by Roy Porter (HarperCollins, 1997); David Higham Associates for an extract from The Body in Question by Jonathan Miller (Jonathan Cape, 1978); Manchester University Press for the extract from The Black Death by Rosemary Horrox (Manchester University Press, 1994).

Every effort has been made to trace and acknowledge ownership of copyright. The publishers will be glad to make suitable arrangements with any copyright holders whom it has not been possible to contact.

Introduction

This book is about how medicine has changed and developed from prehistoric times to today – a period of over 22,000 years!

To help you make sense of all this, these 22,000 years have been divided into the following periods:

- prehistoric   we have evidence for the period 20 000 BC to 3000 BC
- ancient civilisations   The Ancient Egyptians 3000 BC to 500 BC

    The Ancient Greeks 1000 BC to 250 BC

    The Romans 300 BC to 600 AD
- the Middle Ages   400 AD to 1500 AD
- the Renaissance   1500 AD to 1700 AD
- the 18th to 20th centuries
- the 21st century.

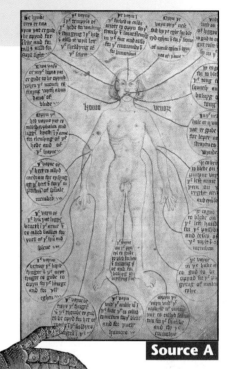

Source A

Study the six pictures on the right. Match each picture to one of these descriptions:

> a medicine man
> the god Asclepios curing a sick woman
> blood-letting
> artificial hands
> the first operation using anaesthetic
> keyhole surgery.

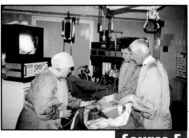

Source C

For each picture:

- match it to one of the periods listed above
- explain whether it shows that people believed disease was caused by supernatural or natural causes.

As you are studying how medicine changed, there are some very important questions that you need to keep in mind. These questions will keep cropping up as you go through this book. By the end of the course you should have developed your own ideas about these questions – and have some examples to support these ideas.

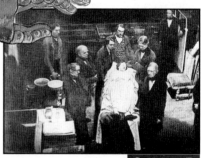

Source B

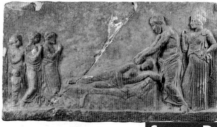

Source D

1 In what ways has medicine changed?
2 How do factors like: chance;

                  individuals;

                  government;

                  religion;

                  war;

                  science and technology;

  bring about change?

3 What different ideas have people had about what causes and cures illness?
4 Why has there been faster change in some periods than in others?
5 Has change always brought benefits?

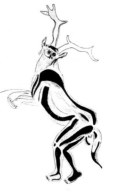

Source F

Source E

How do we know about prehistoric medicine?

For the exam you will need to know:

☑ The difficulties we face in finding evidence about prehistoric medicine

☑ How changing lifestyles affected medicine

☑ Whether prehistoric medicine was based on natural or supernatural ideas and methods.

Prehistoric means before we have written records. We have written records from Egypt around 3000 BC, but before that we have to depend on other types of evidence.

Hunters and gatherers

For about 2.5 million years tool-making people have lived on earth. However, most of the evidence we have about them comes from between 20,000 and 10,000 years ago.

These people were hunters and gatherers. They lived in groups of between 30 and 100.

Life for them was harsh, brutish and often short.

Because they had to keep moving they probably left the sick to die and even killed young babies if there were too many to look after or if they were slowing up the movement of the group.

Archaeological evidence shows they were often deformed, racked with arthritis, and covered with injuries like broken limbs. They had gangrene because bacteria had got into wounds, they caught rabies from animals like wolves and they got infections by eating raw animal flesh.

OISÍN MCGANN 2002

This doesn't sound too good. However, they did not suffer from many of the diseases that are common in the modern world.

■ They were nomads and did not stay in one place long enough to pollute water supplies. They did not pile up filth that attracts disease-carrying insects.

■ Infections like smallpox and measles were almost unknown because the micro-organisms that cause contagious diseases need lots of people living close together to be able to spread.

■ They did not keep cattle or poultry that spread diseases to humans.

■ They ate a wide range of wild plant and animal food which gave them all the nutrients they needed to be healthy.

They suffered badly from organisms like worms and lice.

Farmers

About 12,000 to 10,000 years ago there was a major change. People settled down and started to farm. It is usually said that this was a big step forward for humans – but did it do much for their health?

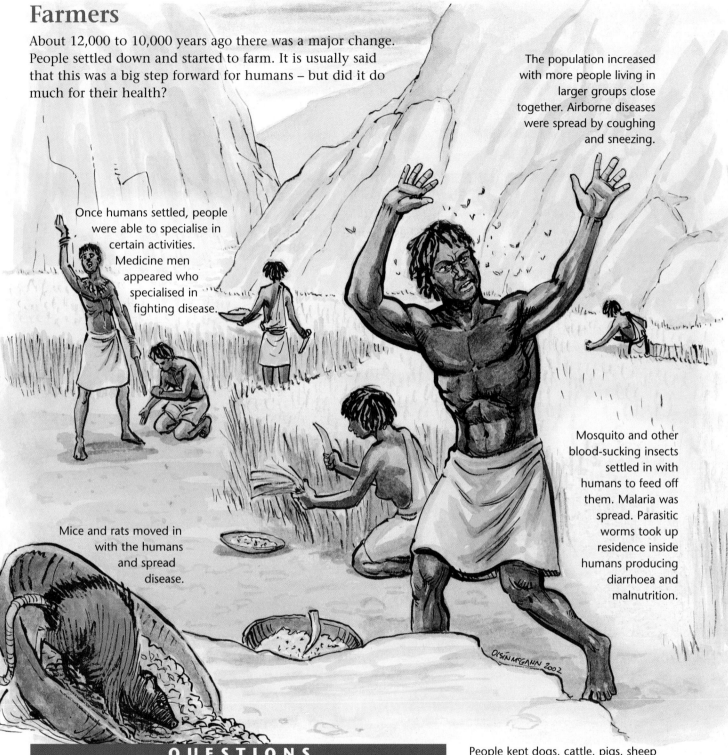

The population increased with more people living in larger groups close together. Airborne diseases were spread by coughing and sneezing.

Once humans settled, people were able to specialise in certain activities. Medicine men appeared who specialised in fighting disease.

Mosquito and other blood-sucking insects settled in with humans to feed off them. Malaria was spread. Parasitic worms took up residence inside humans producing diarrhoea and malnutrition.

Mice and rats moved in with the humans and spread disease.

People kept dogs, cattle, pigs, sheep and poultry. The diseases from these animals spread to humans. Historians have estimated that humans share 65 diseases with dogs and 50 with cattle. These animals spread diseases by fouling drinking water and cultivated land. Polio, cholera and typhoid spread to humans.

QUESTIONS

1   Name four ways in which the change to farming made people unhealthy.

2   Name four ways in which the change to farming made people more healthy.

3   Write three paragraphs explaining how far you agree with the following statement: 'Farming was a healthier lifestyle than hunting and gathering.'

SOURCE INVESTIGATION

What evidence have we got from prehistoric times?

Look at the evidence on these two pages and see what you can work out about the diseases prehistoric people suffered from and the methods they used to treat the sick.

Q1 Draw a chart showing what we can learn under the following headings:

- illnesses they suffered from
- their ideas about what caused illness
- how they treated illnesses and tried to make people better.

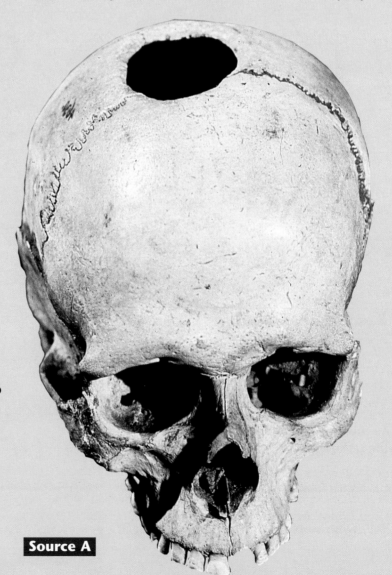

A prehistoric trephined skull. Flint cutting tools were used to scrape away a hole in the skull, often with great skill. This may have been done to release an evil spirit, or to relieve headaches or epilepsy. We know that some patients survived because the bone at the edges of the hole had begun to grow again.

Source A

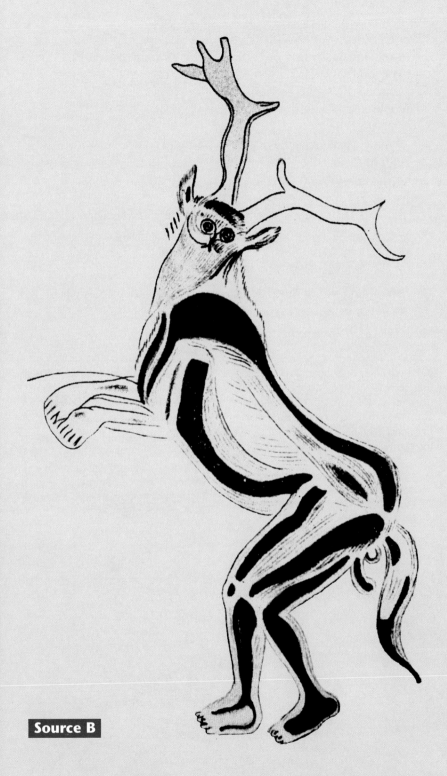

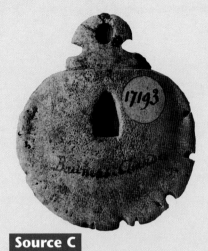

Source C

Bone used as an amulet (a charm worn as a protection against evil spirits).

Source B

A cave painting found in southern France. This is probably the oldest known painting of a Medicine Man. Medicine Men had god-given powers to heal the sick by destroying their enemies using effigies or magic rituals to prevent disease.

As you have seen we have little evidence from prehistoric times. One other way of finding out about prehistoric medicine is to study primitive modern societies. They might still be using the beliefs and methods that were used in prehistoric times.

There are two basic ways to explain illness:

■ natural causes – hunger, climate, accidents, parasites and wounds

■ supernatural causes – spirits of the dead, planets, witches and magic.

Featured on these two pages are some examples of approaches to illness from:

■ the Aborigines of Australia – until recently all their tools were made of stone and wood

■ the Azande of southern Sudan, in Africa.

By a process of observation and trial and error the Aborigines had discovered the use of plants. They also knew that heat helped to relieve pain and swelling. Here are some of the remedies they used:

■ Open cuts were covered with a pad of mud, clay, or animal fat, or closed up with an eaglehawk feather and bound with layers of bark and kangaroo skin.
■ Broken arms were encased in mud and clay.

■ Rheumatic pains, fevers and swellings were treated with steam from a pit of damped grass laid on burning bark.

We now know that many of the herbs and plants used by 'primitive' societies were effective. Some, for example, were antiseptics, others were anaesthetics.

Source D

A description of 20th-century Aborigines.

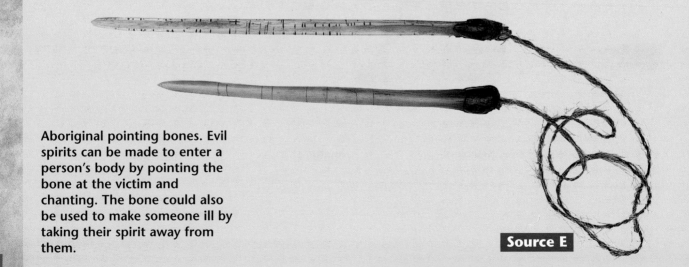

Aboriginal pointing bones. Evil spirits can be made to enter a person's body by pointing the bone at the victim and chanting. The bone could also be used to make someone ill by taking their spirit away from them.

Source E

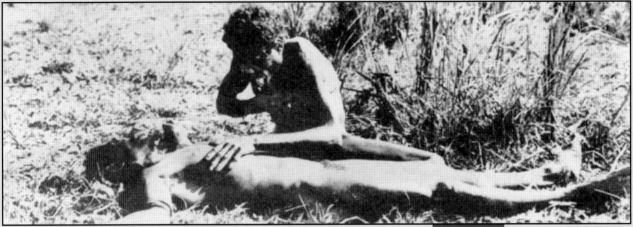

Source F

Whenever members of the tribe fell ill they blamed either witchcraft or sorcery. Witches were born with a 'witch-organ' a large cyst under the liver. They had no control over the evil effects of the organ. Emotions overheated the organ which then made someone ill. Sorcerers, on the other hand, could control their bad magic and deliberately made people ill. The Azande consulted an oracle to find out who was harming them. This was done by giving a chicken poison. It is commanded to die if the person named is guilty.

Source G

A 20th-century description of the Azande.

Q2   From the evidence about the Aborigines and the Azande make a list of natural approaches and a list of supernatural approaches.

Q3   How far does the evidence from recent peoples like the Aborigines and Azande support the evidence we have got from prehistoric times?

Q4   Are there any problems in using peoples like the Aborigines and Azande as evidence about prehistoric medicine?

An Aboriginal Medicine Man massaging a sick man with sweat from his armpits. The Aborigines believed that illness is caused by something evil being introduced into the body by magic. The Medicine Man then sucks the injured part of the body to remove the evil.

The Azande only consult oracles when the illness is serious. In cases of mild illness or injury, the situation is usually treated: an injured foot is bound and poulticed; an abscess will be cleaned and often scalded with hot water.

Source H

A 20th-century description of the Azande.

HELP YOUR REVISION

Factors

■ The lifestyle of prehistoric people affected their health – the change to farming made it easier and harder to stay healthy!

Ideas about causes

■ They believed illness was caused by spirits.

Other important points

■ We have little evidence about prehistoric medicine.

■ For simple wounds or illnesses they used natural treatments.

Ancient Egyptian medicine – natural or supernatural?

For the exam you will need to know:

☑ How we know about Egyptian medicine

☑ Whether religion helped Egyptian medicine

☑ How natural and supernatural ideas existed side by side

☑ How Egyptian doctors worked

☑ The Egyptian theory about how illness is caused.

The period of the great Ancient Egyptian civilisation began around 3000 BC when the two kingdoms of Upper and Lower Egypt were united. It ended in 525 BC when Egypt was conquered by the Persians who were then conquered by the Greek Alexander the Great in 323 BC.

Where was Ancient Egypt?

You might know where Egypt is today. Ancient Egypt was rather different. It was limited to land a few miles either side of the River Nile. To the west and east there was nothing but desert (see Source A).

Factor 1:

The isolation of Ancient Egypt

As you can see the Ancient Egyptians were cut off from other civilisations. This led to long-term stability as they were not being constantly invaded and so could make steady progress in areas like engineering and medicine.

However, their isolation had another result – for most of the period 3000 BC to 300 BC their medicine stayed the same. There were few advances. This was because no new ideas from other countries reached them.

Factor 2:

The River Nile

The River Nile fertilised the land on its banks, but it did more than this. Every summer the river rose by about seven metres. This led to water flooding onto the farming land by the Nile. It also left on the land huge amounts of silt which fertilised the land and made it good for growing crops. Producing enough food was never a problem for the Egyptians. This meant they had plenty of time for other activities like building and medicine.

Factors influencing

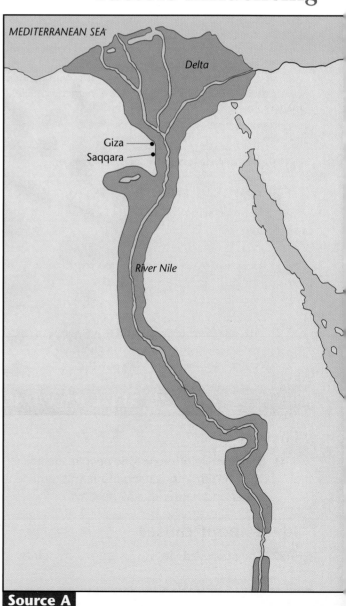

MEDITERRANEAN SEA

Delta

Giza

Saqqara

River Nile

Map of Ancient Egypt

Source A

Factor 3:

Irrigation

The Egyptians built irrigation channels from the Nile to take water to the surrounding land. It was important to keep these channels clear of blockages. If the water did not get through, the land would return to desert and the crops would die. Some historians think that this gave the Egyptians a natural theory about how disease was caused. They knew there were vessels all around the body carrying blood, air and urine. They seem to have thought that disease was caused by these vessels becoming blocked. This led to treatments like blood-letting to clear the blockages. This was the first natural explanation of illness.

Egyptian medicine

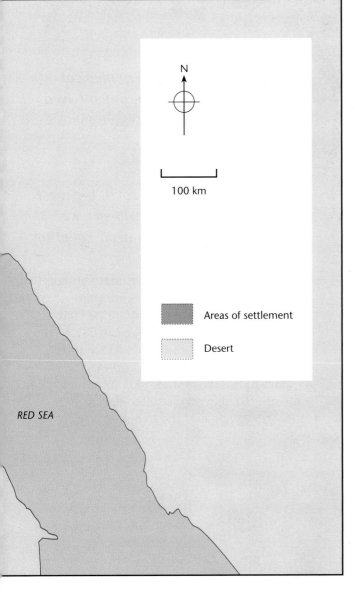

Factor 4:

Hieroglyphics

The Egyptians developed a system of writing using signs called hieroglyphics. This meant they could keep records of illnesses and treatments. This information could be shared with other doctors and handed down to later generations. Gradually they built up a huge bank of knowledge about medicine.

Factor 5:

Religion

Egyptian religious beliefs may have helped them learn about the structure of the human body. They regarded life as a preparation for afterlife. In this afterlife the body and its organs were needed. The liver, lungs, stomach and intestines were taken out, treated with spices to preserve them, and stored in Canopic jars. The brain was removed through the nostrils with hooks, and the body was soaked for 70 days in natron, treated with gums and finally wrapped in long strips of linen. The embalmers who did all this must have learnt a lot about the structure of the body and this knowledge may have been passed on to doctors.

The route for the removal of the brain. The arrows show the bones through which holes had to be made. These were only 2 cm in diameter.

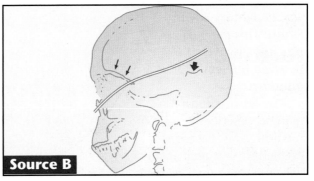

Source B

QUESTIONS

1 From what you have read so far is it likely that the Ancient Egyptians were more advanced in medicine than prehistoric societies? Give three reasons for your answer.

How do we know about Egyptian medicine?

Egyptian papyri.

The Egyptians developed a system of writing using hieroglyphics. Some of these writings have survived but until about 180 years ago nobody could understand them. Even today we cannot understand all the signs.

Writings about medicine were carved on stone or written in ink on papyri (paper made from reeds). These papyri are the most important source of information we have about Egyptian medicine.

The two most famous papyri are the Edwin Smith papyrus (named after the American who bought it in Egypt in 1862) and the Ebers papyrus, also bought by Edwin Smith. This papyrus was first discovered between the legs of a mummy!

The Edwin Smith papyrus describes a series of medical cases. Each one is divided into: *Examination, diagnosis, prognosis and treatment.* They show the careful method used by doctors – very similar to what a doctor does today when a patient visits the surgery. The methods used are free of magic.

We have a few accounts of Egyptian medicine from travellers who visited Egypt.

The Egyptians did leave some drawings about their medicine.

Unfortunately, many of the drawings are of pharaohs who are shown as young with perfect limbs, strong muscles and no fat. Most of the women are tall, slender and beautiful. However, as you will see later, there are a few drawings that are more realistic.

No Egyptian medical equipment has survived – but we do have some drawings of it.

After the papyri, the most important evidence we have is from dead Egyptian bodies!

The dry, hot climate of Egypt means that bodies are well preserved, especially those that were mummified. We can X-ray the bodies, use fibre-optics to see inside them, and take DNA samples. These methods have told us a lot about the diseases the Egyptians suffered, how healthy they were and the treatments they received.

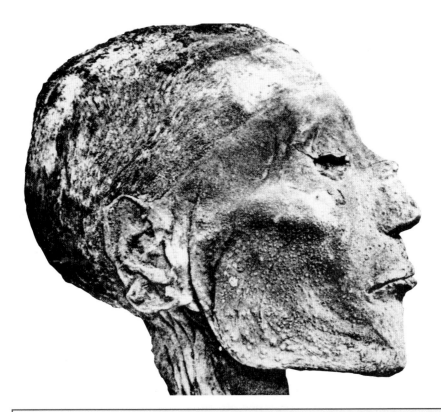

Source A

The mummified face of an Egyptian pharaoh showing traces of disease, probably smallpox.

Case 16 – This account from the Edwin Smith papyrus is so clear and detailed that doctors today can tell this patient suffered from a fracture in the base of the skull and then developed tetanus (lock-jaw). ▼

Instructions for a gaping wound in his head, extending to the bone.

Examination

You should then probe his wound though he shudders greatly. You should then cause him to lift his face. It is painful for him to open his mouth. His heart beats too weakly for speech. You observe his saliva falling from his lips but not falling completely. He discharges blood from his two nostrils and from his two ears. He suffers stiffness in his neck. He does not find he can look at his two shoulders and his breast.

Diagnosis and Prognosis

You shall say concerning him 'one having a gaping wound in his head extending to the bone and penetrating the skull. His muscles are contracted, he discharges blood from his two nostrils and from his two ears; and he suffers from stiffness in his neck.'

Treatment

As soon as you find that his muscles and jaws are contracted, you should make him drink something hot until he is comfortable and his mouth opens. You should then bind it with oil and honey.

Second Examination

If you find his flesh is hot under the wound. That man, he has developed toothache under that wound. You put your hand on him and you find his brow is wet with sweat. The muscles of his neck are taut, his face is flushed. The odour of his head is like the excrement of cattle. He cannot open his mouth, his two eyebrows drawn, his face as if he was weeping.

Second Diagnosis and Prognosis

He has developed toothache; he cannot open his mouth; he suffers stiffness of his neck – an ailment not to be treated.

Third Examination

If you now find that he has become pale and already shows exhausation.

Third Treatment

You should then place in his mouth a wedge of wood, padded with linen. You should then have made for him a drink of almonds. His treatment is sitting down, placed between two supports until there is a development.

Source B

QUESTIONS

1 What are the similarities and differences between the evidence we have about Egyptian medicine and the evidence we have about prehistoric times?

2 What can you learn about Egyptian medicine from Source B?

What can we learn from this evidence about Egyptian medicine?

What did they know about anatomy (the structure of the body)?

Human dissection was not allowed out of respect for the dead. However, doctors had opportunities to observe the human skeleton when treating soldiers wounded in battle, and when bodies were embalmed. The embalmers were very skilful in removing internal organs that would rot (liver, lungs, stomach and intestines) through a small cut in the body. They also removed the brain through the nose (see page 13).

Did doctors learn about the body from the embalmers? We are not sure. Some Egyptian writings tell us that embalmers were regarded as unclean. However, we know from other writings that some doctors were also embalmers. It seems likely that they did learn something.

The Egyptians seem to have had a good knowledge of the structure of the body. They had names for many parts of the body, external and internal. Source A shows the parts of the skull. They also knew about the existence of: veins, arteries, muscles, and a lot about bone structure e.g. the backbone and the ribs. However, their religious beliefs also held them back from making further discoveries. As the body was needed in the afterlife, dissection was forbidden and so doctors had no opportunity to study other parts of the body.

Parts of the skull named by the Egyptians.

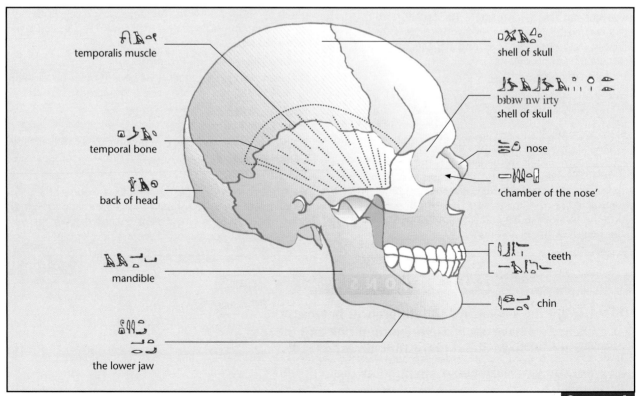

temporalis muscle

temporal bone

back of head

mandible

the lower jaw

shell of skull

bȝbȝw nw irty
shell of skull

nose

'chamber of the nose'

teeth

chin

Source A

What did they know about physiology (how the body works)?

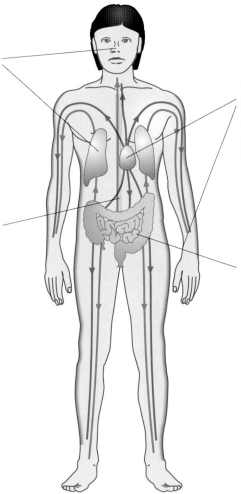

Breathing – they got close to understanding this. They thought air was drawn in through the **nose** into the **lungs**, then to the heart and then to all parts of the body.

They did not know about the circulation of the blood but they did say that the **heart** could speak through the vessels to all limbs. They also felt the **pulse** of patients and knew that a heart beating weakly was a worrying sign (see Source B).

They knew a little about the nervous system e.g. that the **spinal cord** was important for transferring information to the lower part of the body. Notes in a papyrus mention a patient 'not knowing his two legs and his two arms' because of a dislocation of the neck. However, they do not seem to have realised that the brain controlled the rest of the body because they threw it away after it was taken out of the body.

They also believed that diseases were spread to the rest of the body by vessels from the **bowels**.

If any doctor, any priest or any magician places his fingers on the head, on the hands, on the place of the heart, he measures the heart because its speaks out of every limb.

There are: 4 vessels to his two ears.

4 vessels to the liver; it is they which give humour and air, which afterwards cause all diseases in it by overfilling with blood.

4 vessels that open to the anus; it is they which cause humour and air to be produced for it. The anus opens to every vessel in the arms and legs when it is overfilled with excrements.

Source B

From the Ebers papyrus.

QUESTIONS

1 Explain how religion both helped and hindered the Egyptians finding out more about the human body. Overall, did religion help more than it hindered? Give reasons for your answer.

Natural ideas and treatments about the causes of injuries and disease

Source A

This carving comes from the tomb of a worker in a cemetery. It shows how injuries could happen at work. Can you see: the worker dropping his mallet on to another worker's foot; a worker having something removed from his eye; someone having a dislocated shoulder dealt with?

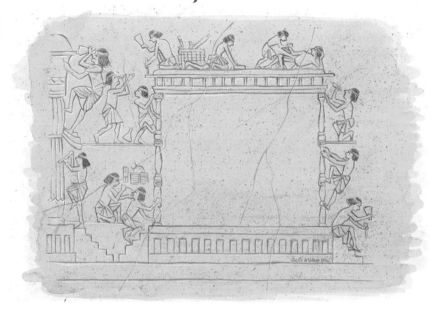

The Egyptians had a good understanding of external injuries like those caused in battle, at work, or by animals. When the cause of the injury was obvious such as in flesh wounds, fractures, bites and stings the Egyptians used natural treatments and did not use magic.

Descriptions in papyri and wall paintings, and the actual mummies themselves, tell us about some of the diseases the Egyptians suffered from. Diseases caused by parasites, especially worms, have been found in mummies. Diseases of the eye were common as were smallpox and plague.

Source B

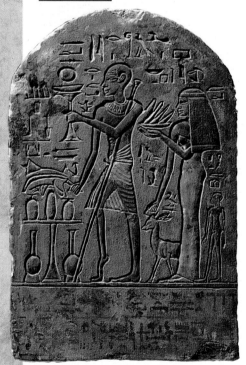

A carving showing a doorkeeper with a shortened and deformed leg. This may have been due to polio.

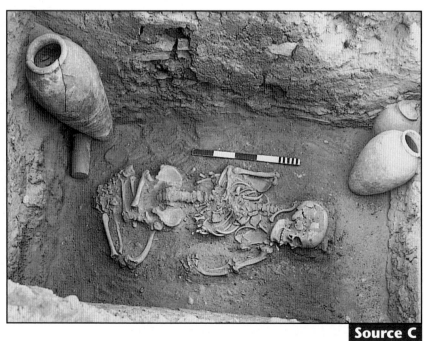

Source C

An Egyptian mummy with dwarfism.

Doctors and their methods

Egyptian doctors had a good reputation and kings of other countries like Persia often used them. Temples often had special schools attached to them where doctors were trained. These temple doctors were paid a salary by the pharaoh and provided free treatment. Ordinary doctors were paid in goods or services.

The papyri (look back at Source B on page 15) show that Egyptian doctors were trained to use an approach which is very similar to what doctors do today!

1 Listen to patients' symptoms then examine them using their eyes and hands

2 Reach their diagnosis and say if the illness can be treated

3 Treat the patient using their experience of patients with similar illnesses.

We know that many doctors were specialists. The Greek traveller Herodotus tells us this in Source D. In Source E you can see funeral inscriptions that tell of the specialities practised by a doctor in the royal palace around 1500 BC. He was called 'Chief Physician' and the fact that his tomb was located near the tomb of a local governor shows he was important.

Many of the treatments used by the Egyptians were drugs prepared from animals, like excrement of crocodile and bile of tortoise, and from over 160 different plants such as barley, grapes, raisins and watermelon. These would be mashed or strained in water, alcohol or oil. They imported many substances from abroad e.g. cinnamon from China and perfumes and spices from Abyssinia. Medicines were given in different forms: as pills, cakes, ointments, drops and baths.

Medicine with them is organised in the following way: every doctor is for one disease and not for several, and the whole country is full of doctors of the eyes; others of the head; others of the teeth; others of the belly, and others of obscure diseases.

Source D

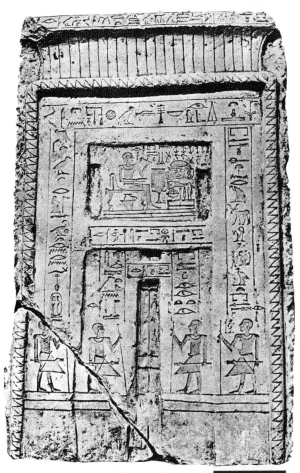

Source E

These inscriptions tell us that Ir-en-akhty was a palace doctor, inspector of the palace doctors, palace ophthalmologist, palace gastroenterologist, guardian of the anus, and palace eye doctor.

Burns –	Day 1	black mud
	Day 2	excrement of cattle, barley dough, oil
	Day 3	barley dough, oil, resin of acacia
	Day 4	wax, oil, cooked unwritten papyrus
	Day 5	red ochre, carob, copper flakes

Source F

Treatment for a burn from the Ebers papyrus.

Another remedy for the belly: almonds, wormwood, sweet beer; made into one thing. It is to cause a man to evacuate all which is in his belly.

Source H

From the Ebers papyrus.

Some of the treatments used by the Egyptians would have been effective:

- rotten bread was used in several treatments and would have been effective on wounds because of the antibacterial moulds
- substances like lead, copper salts and carbon were used for beautifying women's eyes. These substances are antiseptic and would have helped with eye infections which were common in Egypt
- radishes, garlic and onions were fed to workmen building the pyramids. We now know that these contain chemicals effective against dysentery, typhoid and cholera.

When illness was internal the Egyptians had more problems. As we have seen they believed the vessels or channels spread poisonous substances from the bowel which could lead to blockages and cause disease. They tried to clear such blockages by blood-letting, vomiting and by using laxatives like castor oil. Blood-letting was carried out by puncturing the skin or by using leeches.

QUESTIONS

1 Imagine you are an Egyptian doctor. Keep a diary for a week. Make entries in your diary showing what complaints patients came to you with, how you examined them, and what treatments you used.

Surgery

Surgery was not separate from general medicine. It seems to have been practised by all doctors. They only carried out simple operations e.g. cutting out swellings. They certainly did not carry out much surgery – 30,000 mummies have been examined without a single surgical scar being found. No evidence has been found of drugs other than alcohol being used to numb the pain. The Egyptians certainly did not carry out major operations like the Romans.

However, there is evidence that they used hammer and chisel for trephining – to get access to the brain. We know patients survived because of the healing of bone edges.

Wounds were bandaged with fresh meat, then bound with oil and honey – the sugars draw out fluids and reduce the swelling. Bacteria do not grow in honey and so it also helped wounds heal. Excrement, blood, urine, and animal fat were also used for wounds. These were stitched with needles, and bandaging was used to close the wounds. By examining bones we can also tell that fractures were set with splints and healed well.

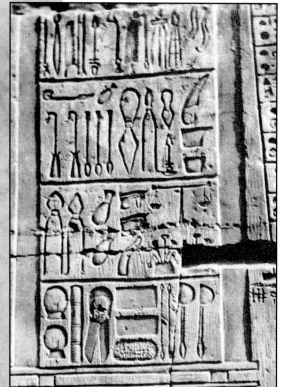

An inscription from a temple wall showing surgical instruments. Can you see the following: a saw, tooth forceps, cupping vessels (for bleeding), sponge, scalpels?

Source A

Instructions for a fracture in the chamber of his nose

Examination

If you examine a man having a fracture in the nose, and you find his face crooked and his face is flat: the swelling which is over it is large.

Diagnosis

Then you shall say 'One suffering from a fracture in the chamber of his nose, an ailment which I will treat.'

Treatment

Clean out what is in his two nostrils with swabs of linen, until every worm of blood in his nostrils comes forth. Now you put two swabs of linen, moistened with oil, in his nostrils [to restore the shape of the nose]. You then bandage the nose. You should treat him afterwards with oil and honey, every day, until he is well.

Source B

From the Edwin Smith papyrus.

QUESTIONS

1 Who was more advanced in surgery: people in prehistoric times or the Ancient Egyptians? Give examples to support your answer.

Herodotus.

Public health

Herodotus called the Egyptians the 'healthiest of all men'. The Egyptians did take great care to keep their bodies and their homes clean. This was probably mainly due to religious reasons. They believed that keeping clean was a way of being at peace with the gods and the spirits. Rich and poor washed every morning, evening, and before each meal. Regular purgings and vomitings were just as important as they cleansed the insides of the body. However, it is important to remember that it was the responsibility of each individual to keep clean; the Egyptian government did not provide a public health system to help everyone keep clean.

They are especially religious and these are some of their customs:
They drink from cups of bronze which they clean daily and this is done by everyone. They are especially careful always to wear newly washed linen clothing. Their priests shave the whole body every third day so that no lice may infest them while they are in the service of the gods. Twice a day and every night all Egyptians wash in cold water.

Source C

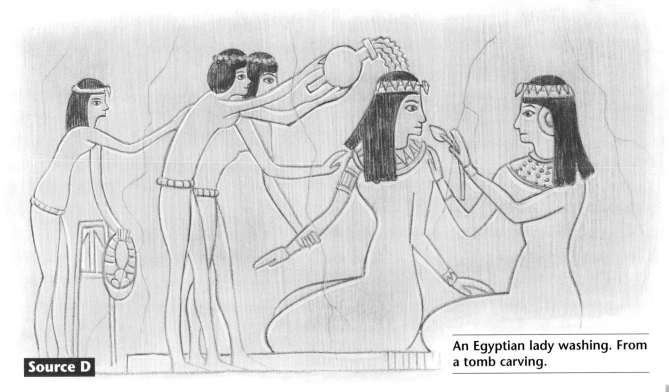

Source D

An Egyptian lady washing. From a tomb carving.

Magic and religion

We have seen that the Egyptians had proper doctors and natural treatments for illness – so why did they also turn to magic and religion?

- Supernatural influences were major controlling factors in the everyday life of the Egyptians. Gods controlled everything including the movement of the stars, the flooding of the Nile and disease. Gods were such an everyday part of life it was natural to turn to them when you were ill.

- Doctors who worked in temples would also be priests. To them it was natural to use both natural and supernatural methods.

- Doctors were expensive and their treatments were often painful.

- There was no certainty that the doctor's treatments would work – and they often did not, whereas magic and religion did sometimes work because patients believed they were going to get better.

- With external injuries the cause was often obvious and a natural treatment was to hand, but the Egyptians did not know the causes of internal injuries or of diseases – this is when they turned to the gods. They did not know about bacteria entering the body from outside and causing infection. Instead, they believed in evil spirits entering the body from outside.

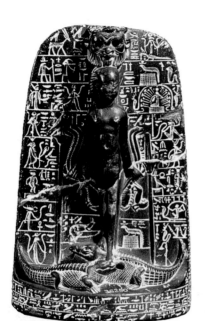

Source A

A stone carving believed to give protection from attack by animals like snakes. It shows Horus having control over poisonous animals. The head of Bes is at the top for extra protection.

It is important to remember that the Egyptians found nothing strange in using natural and supernatural methods alongside each other. They did not make the distinction between these methods that we make today.

Gods like Osiris and Horus protected humans from disease or healed them. Pregnant women prayed to the god Bes, while Thoth was the most important healing god. Temples and shrines were built for the worship of these gods. Gods like Seth brought disease to humans by sending demons to enter the body.

The Egyptians called on the help of the gods by saying spells like this one for a snake bite: 'Flow out poison. Come forth. Go forth on to the ground. Horus will exorcise you. He will punish you. He will spit you out.'

Some spells combined magic with natural treatments: 'To be recited when medicine is drunk – I have utterances that the lord of the universe has composed to kill the doings of a god, a goddess, that are in this my head, in these my bones, in these my shoulders, in these my limbs.'

The love poem in Source B also shows this combined approach of natural and supernatural.

It is seven days from yesterday since I saw my love,
And sickness has crept over me,
My limbs have become heavy,
I cannot feel my own body.
If the master-doctors come to me
I gain no comfort from their remedies.
And the priest-magicans have no cures.

Written in about 1500 BC.

Source B

Another way to use magic was to wear an amulet (an object worn as protection against evil). These were very popular. They were worn by the living and buried with the dead. Some had drawings of animals that, for example, had good eyesight or strong hearts, others had drawings of gods like Bes on them.

Gods like Imhotep had healing centres built alongside their temples. Here patients were immersed in healing holy water or slept overnight in hope of having a dream in which a god would indicate a cure.

QUESTIONS

1 Draw a table with two headings: supernatural medicine and natural medicine. In the column under each heading write down five examples.

HELP YOUR REVISION

Factors

- They made progress because they were settled, and they had writing.
- Their isolation prevented them from making more progress.
- Did their religion help or hinder progress?

Ideas about disease

- Gods cause disease.
- They had a natural theory about illness being caused by channels in the body becoming blocked.

Other important points

- Supernatural and natural beliefs went side by side.
- They did only simple surgery.
- They took care to keep clean but they did not have a public health system.
- They had some understanding of the anatomy and physiology of the body.
- Doctors developed a method of examination, diagnosis, prognosis and treatment.

EXAM PRACTICE QUESTIONS

(a) Explain why the Egyptians were able to make progress in medicine.

(b) In which area of medicine did the Egyptians make the most progress?

(c) 'The Egyptians did not think it strange to use supernatural and natural approaches side by side.' How far do you agree with this statement? Explain your answer.

Why were the Greeks able to make so much progress?

For the exam you will need to know:

☑ About Asclepius and temple medicine

☑ The Theory of the Four Humours

☑ Hippocrates and the clinical method of observation

☑ How the Greek philosophers helped the development of medicine

☑ What areas of medicine the Greeks made less progress in.

By 1000 BC the first Greek communities were emerging. By 750 BC cities were built which became independent city states but shared the same language and gods.

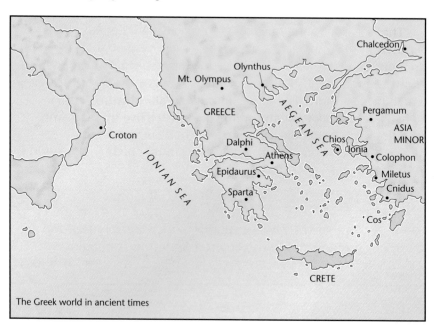

The Greek world in ancient times

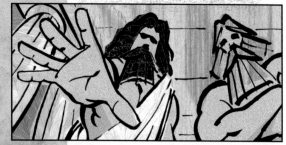

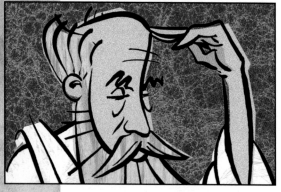

Although they got drugs from the Egyptians the Greeks learned little about medicine from them. Most of their ideas were their own, but like the Egyptians the Greeks mixed supernatural and natural approaches.

Greek medicine can be divided into two traditions:

■ temple medicine and the god Asclepios

■ Hippocrates' Writings and the Theory of the Four Humours.

These two traditions – one mainly supernatural, the other based on natural explanations – survived quite happily side by side in Ancient Greece.

This timeline shows how supernatural and natural ideas existed along side each other in Greek and into Roman times.

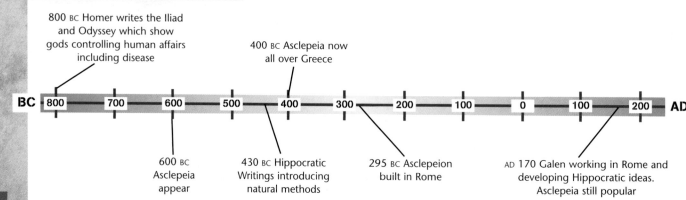

800 BC Homer writes the Iliad and Odyssey which show gods controlling human affairs including disease

400 BC Asclepeia now all over Greece

| BC | 800 | 700 | 600 | 500 | 400 | 300 | 200 | 100 | 0 | 100 | 200 | AD |

600 BC Asclepeia appear

430 BC Hippocratic Writings introducing natural methods

295 BC Asclepeion built in Rome

AD 170 Galen working in Rome and developing Hippocratic ideas. Asclepeia still popular

Asclepios

Much of Greek medicine was based on religion and the belief that the world was controlled by the gods. Apollo was the god of healing, but it is his son Asclepios who became much more important. The Greeks claimed that he was a great doctor who after his death became a god. By 200 BC the cult of Asclepios had spread all over Greece and every large town had a temple to the god called an Asclepeion.

The temples were built on sites of great beauty with pure spring water and refreshing breezes. They were famous as places for cures but also became centres for many other activities.

In fact, an Asclepeion was a combination of a religious shrine and a health resort. The most famous was at Epidauros, near Athens. It was big enough for 500 patients to live there at any one time and had a theatre seating 20,000 people.

A painting from 450 BC showing the gods Apollo and Artemis shooting arrows that brought disease to humans.

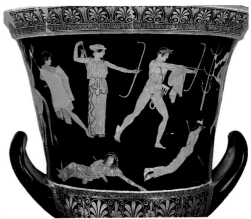

Source A

Artist's impression of an Asclepeion.

Source B

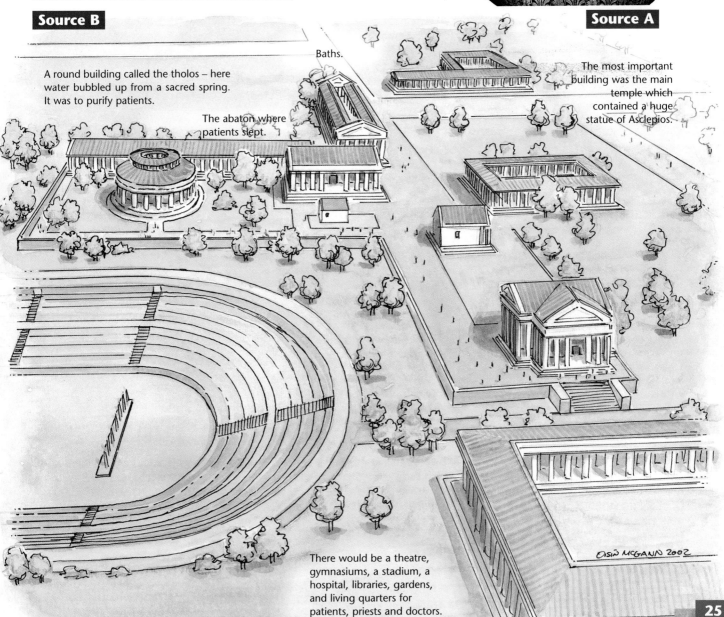

Baths.

A round building called the tholos – here water bubbled up from a sacred spring. It was to purify patients.

The abaton where patients slept.

The most important building was the main temple which contained a huge statue of Asclepios.

There would be a theatre, gymnasiums, a stadium, a hospital, libraries, gardens, and living quarters for patients, priests and doctors.

OISIN McGANN 2002

Visiting an Asclepeion

When you first arrived you would sacrifice an animal to an enormous statue of Asclepios.

You would then be made pure by a series of baths and by going without food and wine.

You would then take part in a series of religious ceremonies and finally be taken into the abaton where you would sleep through the night in full sight of a great statue of the god. You would sleep on beds covered with the skins of animals sacrificed to Asclepios.

While you were asleep the god, with the help of a snake, and his daughters Hygeia and Panacea, would either cure you or would give you a dream. This dream would tell the priests what treatment to use on you.

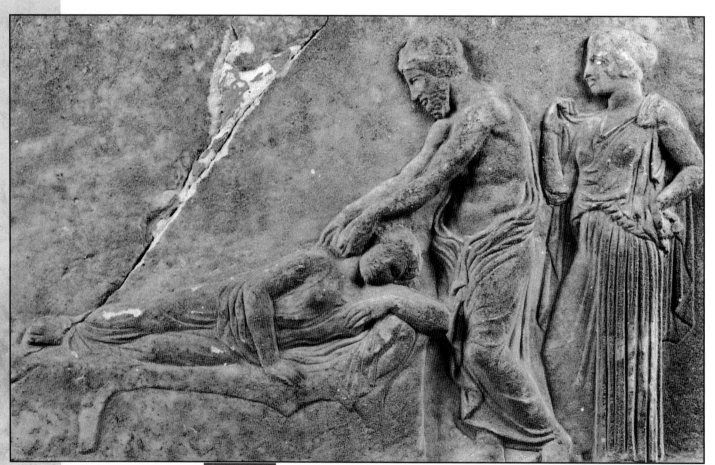

Source A

A carving from a votive from the fourth century BC. It shows Asclepios, helped by Hygeia, treating a sleeping woman.

From a play by Aristophanes about 400 BC. It is about the blind Plutus who visits an Asclepeion to regain his sight.

Asclepios did his rounds, inspecting every patient. He sat down by Plutus and his servant brought him his medicine chest. Asclepios first wiped Plutus' head and then wiped his eyelids with a clean linen cloth. Then Panacea wrapped his head in a purple blanket. Asclepios whistled and two enormous serpents appeared. They glided under the blanket and licked Plutus' eyelids. Plutus sat up and was able to see but the god and his helpers had disappeared.

Source B

The temples mixed the supernatural with natural cures like good diet, rest, massage, bathing and exercise. The priests often used ordinary treatments like bleeding. We know that some of the patients got better because they left behind them inscriptions on stones thanking the god for curing them. Many of these votive stones have been discovered by archaeologists – like Source D.

> Agestratos was unable to sleep because of headaches. As soon as he came to the abaton he fell asleep and had a dream. He thought that the god cured him of his headache and, making him stand up, taught him wrestling. The next day he departed cured, and after a short time he completed at the Namean games and was victor in the wrestling.

Source C

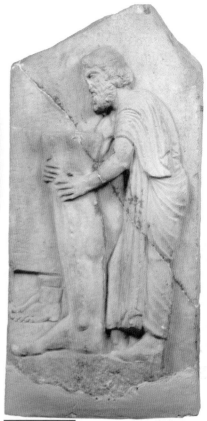

Source D

A votive tablet dedicated to Asclepios, probably for relief from varicose veins.

Why were many of the patients cured? There are several possible explanations.

- Firstly, a lot was due to faith healing. The people visiting the temple genuinely believed in Asclepios' powers and their faith that he would cure them would sometimes lead to them being cured!

- Secondly, when we look at the votive stones we see that many of the people cured were suffering from complaints caused by stress, like headaches, or blindness, caused by some kind of emotional shock. The rest, the good diet, the peace and quiet, the bathing and massage, the escape from the stresses and strains of normal life must have helped these people. So much so that some people stayed for months!

- Finally, we must not forget that the priest did treat the patients using natural methods. Over time they learned a lot about illness and some of their treatments would have worked. So Asclepeia were not just about supernatural medicine.

QUESTIONS

1 Design a poster advertising an Asclepeion.

2 'Asclepeia were only about treating patients by supernatural methods.' Explain whether you agree or disagree with this statement.

Biography

Hippocrates was born about 460 BC on the island of Cos. He died about 370 BC. We know little about him. He was a teacher on Cos and a doctor. He travelled treating patients. He probably wrote some of the books in the Hippocratic collection but we do not know which ones. Somehow the whole collection came to be named after him!

These writings represent a very important step forward in medicine. However, it is important to remember that they were written over a period of hundreds of years and they really represent a gradual development.

Hippocrates' Writings and the Theory of the Four Humours

Gradually some of the priests from Asclepeia began to concentrate more on medicine rather than religion. They had learned a lot about illnesses and treatments and began to move from one town to another treating the sick. Their experiences and their knowledge were finally collected together in the great library of Alexandria around 280 BC. This collection of about 130 books is called the Hippocratic Writings.

Why were the Greeks able to make such advances?

The Greek philosophers

The Greeks were very interested in the natural world in which they lived. They wanted to find out how it worked. Greek philosophers tried to do this by careful observation of everything around them and by lots of hard thinking. By the sixth century BC they agreed that:

- all substances were made from four basic elements: water (wet), earth (dry), fire (hot) and air (cold)
- everything, including the universe and the human body, needed to be kept in balance
- the world can be explained by natural explanations rather than by thinking that the gods controlled everything.

These ideas influenced Greek thinking about medicine. The Hippocratic Writings are important because they include:

- a natural explanation of the causes of disease (the Theory of the Four Humours)
- natural ways of treating patients
- instructions about how doctors should examine their patients (clinical observation)
- the standards by which doctors should do their job (the Hippocratic Oath).

Many of these ideas are just as important today as when they were first developed in Greek times! In fact, we can say that this is when modern medicine begins.

However, the Hippocratic Writings can be criticised because:

- they tell us little about anatomy and physiology
- they say little about surgery
- many of the ideas could only be followed if you were rich. The writings do little to improve the health of the poor.

Illness has natural causes and treatments

The basic idea in the Hippocratic Writings is that everything to do with the human body – health and illness – can be explained naturally. There is no need of supernatural explanations. All disease can be treated by natural treatments e.g. surgery, drugs or diet.

The clinical method of observation

The writings insist that patients must be carefully observed and the findings recorded, turning doctors away from being Medicine Men and miracle healers into the doctors we know today. You will see that the emphasis was on studying the patient rather than the disease; it also concentrated on the whole patient – lifestyle such as diet, work, exercise, sleep, environment – an approach that today's doctors are being encouraged to return to.

The doctor should:

- ask about the patient's past and present behaviour e.g. way of life, work, diet, exercise

- ask the patient about symptoms

- examine the patient carefully: listen to the breathing, take the pulse, take note of any smells, examine body and any excretions

- ignore nothing

- make a record of everything.

> Epilepsy is not any more divine [caused by gods] than other diseases are; there are natural signs that precede the start of the disease. Men believe it is a divine disease because of their ignorance.
>
> **Source A**

Hippocratic Writings: The Sacred Disease.

> The doctor should look at the patient's face. If he looks his usual self this is a good sign. If not, the following are bad signs: a sharp nose, hollow eyes, collapsed temples, cold ears, dry skin on the forehead, the colour of the whole face being green, black or lead-coloured. The doctor must ask if the patient has not been able to sleep, if his bowels have been very loose, or if he has not been eating.
>
> **Source B**

From the Hippocratic Writings: Prognostics.

1st day	He was seized with fever. He had a pain in his head and then became deaf. No sleep, bad fever, tongue dry.
2nd day	Became delirious.
6th day	All the symptoms became worse.
11th day	Constipated. Urine thin and coloured with substances scattered throughout it.
17th day	Swellings about both ears. Legs painful. No sleep.
31st day	Diarrhoea with large discharges of watery matters. Urine thick. Swelling around the ears gone.

Source C

From Hippocratic Writings: Epidemics.

The Hippocratic Writings describe in detail the illnesses of over 40 patients. From these, Greek doctors could build up records of the ways in which different illnesses developed. This would help them to decide what the illness was and what would be suitable treatments.

The writings go on to say: 'It is an excellent thing for a doctor to forecast. If he knows what the next symptoms are likely to be, he can give the patient the right treatment.'

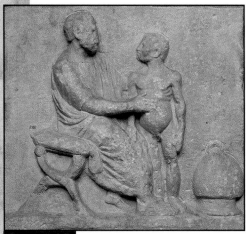

Source A

The tombstone of the Greek doctor Jason (second century BC). He is examining the patient using Hippocratic methods. On the right you can see a bleeding cup. These were heated and placed over a scratch made on the patient's back. As the cup cooled, it drew off a small amount of blood.

The Hippocratic Oath

You can see from the methods used by Hippocratic doctors that they concentrated on understanding the patient as much as the illness. The patient was the key to finding out what was wrong. This concentration on the patient was reflected in the rules for doctors that were laid down in the Hippocratic Oath. This oath set the standards of behaviour for doctors not just in Greek times but for thousands of years afterwards. The oath was taken by medical students in Britain until recently and is still used in many other parts of the world. It could be adapted to Christian times very easily by replacing the Greek gods by God, Christ and the saints. Parts of it, such as the ban on abortion, were particularly attractive to the Christian Church.

Doctors had to swear:

I swear by Apollo, Asclepius and Hygeia and Panacea and all the gods and goddesses, that I will fulfil to my ability and judgement this oath.

Extracts from the Oath:

- I will use my power to help the sick to the best of my ability. I will not harm any man.

- I will not give a deadly drug to anyone. Neither will I help a woman to have an abortion.

- I will not use the knife, but will leave this to those men who do this work.

- Whenever I go into a house, I will go to help the sick and never with the intention of doing harm. I will not indulge in sexual relations with the bodies of men or women.

- Whatever I see or hear, in the course of treating patients, I will keep secret and tell no one.

QUESTIONS

1 You have the job of training Greek doctors. You want to give them a list of the ten most important points they should remember. Make a list of these ten points. Choose two of them and explain why they are important.

2 Find three similarities and three differences between Egyptian and Greek doctors. Who was the more advanced?

The Theory of the Four Humours

The following source is one of the most important sections of the Hippocratic Writings. It describes the Theory of the Four Humours.

Hippocratic Writings: On the Constitution of Man.

Concerning the parts of man's body, it has blood, phlegm, yellow bile and black bile. Through these parts he feels illness or enjoys health. When all of these elements are truly balanced, he feels the most perfect health. Illness occurs when one of these elements is in excess or is lessened in amount. When one of these elements is not balanced by one of the others, the part of the body where it is supposed to make balance naturally becomes diseased.

Source B

This theory was how the Greeks explained the causes of illness. Here it is in the form of a diagram.

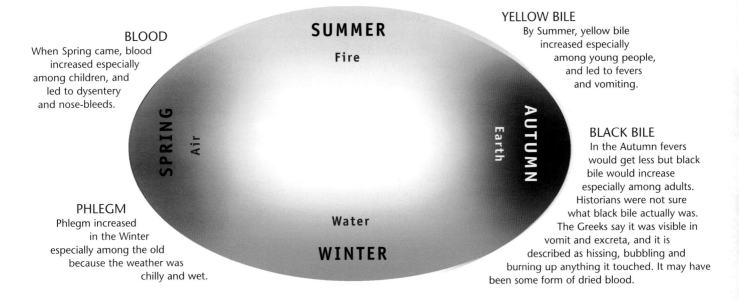

BLOOD
When Spring came, blood increased especially among children, and led to dysentery and nose-bleeds.

YELLOW BILE
By Summer, yellow bile increased especially among young people, and led to fevers and vomiting.

PHLEGM
Phlegm increased in the Winter especially among the old because the weather was chilly and wet.

BLACK BILE
In the Autumn fevers would get less but black bile would increase especially among adults. Historians were not sure what black bile actually was. The Greeks say it was visible in vomit and excreta, and it is described as hissing, bubbling and burning up anything it touched. It may have been some form of dried blood.

SUMMER
Fire
SPRING
Air
AUTUMN
Earth
Water
WINTER

You can see how this theory is a development of the idea of the Greek philosophers that the universe is made up of four basic elements – earth, air, water and fire. In the human body these become cold, dry, moist and hot humours – blood is hot and moist, phlegm is cold and moist, yellow bile is hot and dry, black bile is cold and dry. These humours are normally in balance – this means the person will be healthy. However, when this balance is upset the result is illness.

You will see later that this theory dominated medical thinking for thousands of years. However, some historians think it is the weakest part of the Hippocratic Writings. This is because it confuses causes and results. We know that phlegm, for example, is a result of someone being ill. The Greeks thought it was a cause. You can see why they thought this – when someone is ill they might cough up phlegm or vomit.

Important facts about the Four Humours that you need to know!

What made humours increase and become out of balance with the others? Each humour had its quality e.g. phlegm was cold, so this would increase in the cold of winter. Eating too much could also upset the balance, or not taking enough exercise. The idea of the Four Humours is based on the idea of balance – if anything is done in excess, whether it be eating or exercising, the balance is upset.

QUESTIONS

1 Why do you think the Greeks believed in the Theory of the Four Humours?

Natural treatments

According to Hippocrates the job of the doctor was to help keep the humours in balance. This meant concentrating on the lifestyle of the patient – diet, sleep, exercise.

This could mean:

- blood-letting
- vomiting
- eliminating blood-rich foods like red meat
- encouraging a balanced diet
- encouraging a sensible amount of exercise, bathing, sleep and even sex!

The doctor gently helped nature to restore the balance. Hippocratic doctors believed that doctors should not interfere too much. They believed that nature would eventually put the humours back into balance and the job of the doctor was to help nature a little. They were not keen on using drugs but used gentle drinks like barley water, and honey and water, to keep up the fluid intake. They regarded surgery as an inferior trade because it involved manual work rather than thinking. Even blood-letting was not used much and when it was, bleeding cups were used rather than opening veins with a knife.

Greek doctors also encouraged a lifestyle that would keep the humours in balance – prevention rather than cure. Sport was an important part of Greek life and stadiums and gymnasiums were built all over Greece. It was an important part of the education of boys between the ages of 6–14.

I think that barley soup is better than all other cereal foods for chest diseases – also vinegar and honey for they bring up phlegm and quench thirst.

Source A

Hippocratic Writings – On the Treatment for Acute Diseases.

Keeping healthy begins with the moment a man wakes up. After awakening he should not arise at once but should wait until the heaviness of sleep has gone. After arising he should rub the whole body with some oil. Thereafter he should every day, wash face and eyes with the hands using pure water. He should rub his teeth inside and outside with the fingers using some peppermint powder and cleaning the teeth of remants of food. He should anoint nose and ears inside with well-perfumed oil. He should rub and anoint his head every day but wash it and comb it only at intervals.

A young or middle-aged man should take a walk of about ten stadia just before sunrise. Long walks before meals clear out the body, prepare it for receiving food and give it more power for digesting.

Source B

From the writings of Diocles, a doctor who lived later than Hippocrates, but whose ideas were the same as Hippocrates'.

What weren't the Greeks good at?

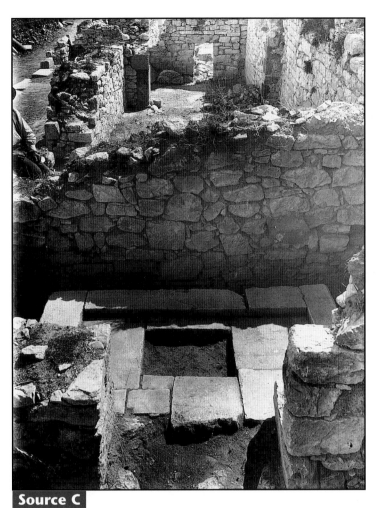

Source C

Rare Greek public lavatories in the Greek city of Corinth (fourth century BC). Continuous running water under the seats took the waste away.

Public health and hygiene

An important point about Greek medicine needs to be made here! Only the rich could afford the time to live the kind of life described in Source C. The rich also had bath tubs and lavatories in their houses which were built in the healthiest and most spacious areas of the city. But what about everyone else? What about the poor, and the slaves?

One visitor to Athens in the third century BC tells us 'Athens has a poor water supply and is badly divided into streets. Its houses are so cheap that a stranger would hardly believe it was the famous city of Athens'. For most people in Greek cities housing was cramped, poorly ventilated, and little better than hovels. The streets were narrow and covered in filth. So much so that all Greeks would wash their feet before entering their homes. Inside, they would have to use wash basins for bathing.

Although many Greeks attempted to keep clean, the city authorities did little to provide public health facilities, to clean the streets, to provide clean water for everyone. The reality of life for many people in the Greek city was rather different from the impression we get from the Hippocratic Writings.

Anatomy and physiology

The Hippocratic Writings have surprisingly little to say about anatomy or physiology. The main organs of the body are described but there is no attempt to give an overall description of the human body. Human dissection was banned and so the Hippocratic writers would have depended entirely on animal dissection, observing wounds, and by looking at what went in, and what came out of, the body!

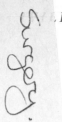

Surgery

Although the Hippocratic doctors looked down on surgery, there are several books about it in the writings so they recognised that it was sometimes necessary. However, they were clear that it was not their job to do it. They regarded surgeons as distinct from, and inferior to, doctors.

- Treatments for fractures and dislocations are mentioned. Splints and bandages were used, and they knew that wounds should be kept dry.

- They also squeezed out pus because they realised it was harmful.

- Simple internal operations were carried out like cutting out tumours and ulcers.

- Cauterisation is mentioned several times: 'What drugs fail to cure, that the knife cures; what the knife cures not, that the fire cures; but what fire fails to cure, this must be called incurable.'

- Some advice is given about operating on patients e.g. on how to prepare the patient, and the lighting and instruments to be used.

Overall, we have to conclude that the Greeks had less interest in, and made less progress in, anatomy, physiology and surgery, than in developing ideas about the causes of disease and how doctors should treat their patients.

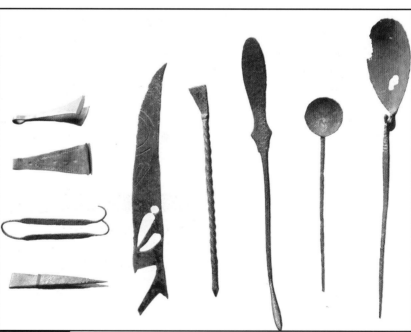

Greek medical instruments.

Source D

Alexandria

Between 336 and 323 BC Alexander the Great made many conquests for the Greeks. One of the areas conquered was Egypt. One of Alexander's generals, Ptolemy, who ruled Egypt for a time made Alexandria his capital and established a great centre of learning there. He built up a massive library, and research into, and teaching of, mathematics, zoology, medicine and many other areas was carried out.

Here Greek doctors were able to carry out human dissections. They were influenced by the ideas of philosophers like Plato and Aristotle who argued that the body is not important after death because only the person's spirit lives on.

Erasistratus dissected the brain and began to understand that the brain sends messages through the nerves to all parts of the body. He also began to describe the structure of the brain and the heart.

This increased knowledge of the body allowed the Greeks to do more surgery and advances were made in the development of surgical instruments. They even began to dissect the eye.

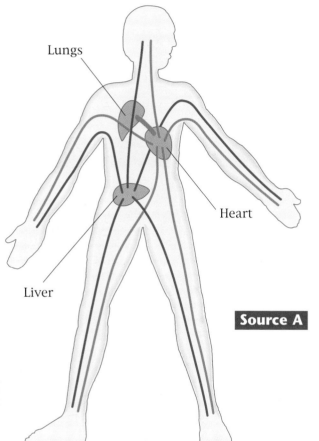

Lungs

Heart

Liver

Source A

Erasistratus realised the heart was a kind of pump. He thought that pneuma (a life-giving substance) was piped to the heart from the lungs. The heart pumped it through the arteries to give life to all parts of the body. (Erasistratus had noticed that the heart sends pulses to the arteries.) Meanwhile blood was formed in the liver and carried by the veins to all parts of the body.

QUESTIONS

1 Greek medicine has some strengths and some weaknesses. What do you think are its three most important strengths? What are its three most important weaknesses?

QUESTIONS

1 Look at the following list. For each item in the list decide if the Egyptians and Greeks had a similar, or a different, approach. Then explain your decision.

Egyptians and Greeks – similarities and differences

Used natural and supernatural approaches side by side	Similar or different? Explain!
Developed a proper method for doctors	Similar or different? Explain!
Found out a lot about anatomy and physiology	Similar or different? Explain!
Developed a natural explanation of the causes of disease	Similar or different? Explain!

HELP YOUR REVISION

Factors

- How did the Greek philosophers help Greek medicine?
- Did religion help or hinder?
- Hippocrates is our first important individual!

Ideas about disease

- Gods cause disease.
- The Theory of the Four Humours.

Other important points

- The Temples of Asclepios.
- They used natural and supernatural approaches side by side.
- They believed in doctors treating the whole patient.
- They laid down a code of conduct for doctors.
- They did not make much progress in anatomy, physiology or surgery.

EXAM PRACTICE QUESTIONS

(a) Explain the Theory of the Four Humours.

(b) Did religion help or hinder progress in medicine in Greek times?

(c) Why were the Greeks able to make more progress in medicine than the Egyptians?

What did the Romans contribute to medicine?

The Romans copy the Greeks!

From 250 BC the Greek world fell more and more under the control of the Roman Empire. By 146 BC Rome controlled much of the Greek world. This had an unexpected effect because it allowed Greek doctors, ideas and gods to make their way into Rome and the Roman Empire.

Asclepios

The Romans borrowed gods from many of the peoples they conquered, including the Greeks. The first temple to Asclepios in Rome was built in 295 BC. Rome was suffering from a terrible plague and the Romans asked the priests at the Greek Asclepeion at Epidaurus for help. Roman legend says that the snake of Asclepios arrived by boat. The temple was built on the spot where the snake landed on the island in the River Tiber. Source A is a Roman coin from about 290 BC showing the arrival of the snake. The temple was still thriving 350 years later. Temples to Asclepios were built throughout the Roman Empire and statues and carvings of the god have even been found in Britain.

For the exam you will need to know:

☑ How the Romans were influenced by the Greeks

☑ Why Galen is important

☑ Why the Romans were able to develop a public health system

☑ What developments the Romans made in surgery

☑ Criticisms of Roman medicine.

Source A

A Roman coin from about 290 BC.

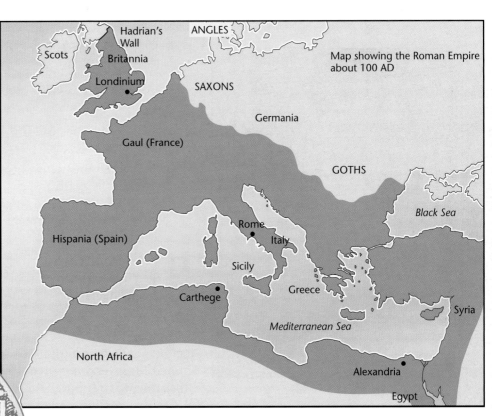

Map of Roman Empire.

Source B

Greek doctors

Most Romans did not think they needed doctors. The head of each household looked after his family's health through the use of charms, prayers and herbs. Upper class Romans would not have dreamt of becoming doctors. The doctor's work was manual and therefore beneath them. There were people practising medicine but they were a motley collection of slaves, root-gatherers, body-builders and schoolteachers all claiming they could treat the sick.

Romans regarded themselves as strong, fit and healthy. They did not need doctors like the weak and feeble Greeks did!

Their approach to medicine was a no-nonsense one and they did not like the fancy theories the Greek doctors were always coming up with. Cicero summed up the Roman approach in the first century BC (see Source B).

However, the influence of Greek ideas on the Romans gradually increased. Greek became the language of the rich and educated, their children were taught by Greek tutors and much of the medicine practised in Rome was Greek. By 80 BC Greek doctors were common in Rome. This was mainly due to Asclepiades (120–70 BC) a Greek doctor who became very popular in Rome and made Greek doctors respectable.

Asclepiades rejects Hippocrates

- Asclepiades rejected Hippocrates' idea that nature only needed a little help from doctors. He claimed that doctors should treat their patients more.

- He dismissed the idea that the body is made up of Four Humours.

- He claimed the human body is made of atoms always moving through the pores and channels of the body. Between these atoms flowed the body liquids. Health depended on the atoms and liquids moving smoothly and this depended on getting a balance between relaxation and tension through diet, exercise, massage and cold water bathing.

- He also supported bleeding, and cutting down on food and drink during fevers. However these treatments just made the patients weaker.

The popularity of Asclepiades had two results: (i) it made Greek doctors popular, and (ii) it meant that Hippocrates' ideas were ignored for several hundreds of years. It would take Galen, another Greek doctor, to bring them back into popularity.

The Romans still had mixed feelings about Greek doctors. Many resented the influence Greek ideas had and preferred the more down-to-earth Roman approach.

Source D shows you what Pliny the Elder had to say about Greek doctors in the first century BC.

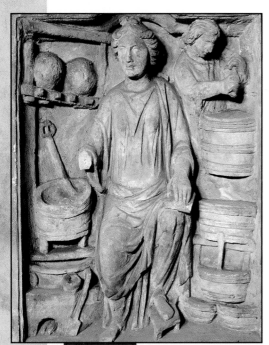

Source C

A Roman carving showing a woman pharmacist. There were also female midwives and doctors.

Why were Greek doctors mistrusted?

- They were foreigners.

- The Romans had conquered the Greeks and so saw them as inferior.

- Greek doctors were always disagreeing with each other about illness and how to treat it (e.g. Asclepiades rejected Hippocrates' ideas).

- Some patients treated by Greek doctors did die!

However, we should not think that Pliny represented the views of all Romans and many wealthy families employed Greek doctors in their households. In 46 BC Julius Caesar passed a law allowing doctors to become citizens of Rome, and 200 years later laws were passed controlling the training of doctors.

Ideas about medicine

The Romans were not interested in thinking about the causes of disease. Nor did they add many new ideas about treatments. If you read Source E, you will probably think this was just as well.

They depended on the Greeks for ideas about anatomy, causes of disease and how to treat patients. This brings us to Galen who you will read about next.

> There is no doubt that they all risk our lives, in order to be the discoverer of some new thing to win reputations for themselves. Hence too that gloomy inscription on monuments 'It was the crowd of doctors which killed me.' There is alas no law against incompetency. They learn by putting us in danger and make experiments until their patients die, and the doctor is the only person not punished for murder.

Source D

> Sores, burns, anal trouble, cracked skin and scorpion bites are also treated with urine. The greatest midwives say that no better washing material exists for skin diseases. Urine cures head wounds, dandruff and sores on the genitals. Every individual benefits most from his own urine. A dog-bite should immediately be washed with urine.

Source E

From 'The Blessing of Urine' by Pliny the Elder, in the first century AD.

QUESTIONS

1 Did Greek ideas help or hinder the development of Roman medicine?

2 'The Roman approach to medicine was the same as the Greeks'.' From what you know so far explain whether you agree or disagree with this statement.

Galen the showman

It is possible to argue that Galen is the most important person you will read about in this book. He rescued the ideas and methods of Hippocrates (which had been rejected by Asclepiades), and made many discoveries of his own which took Hippocrates' ideas further. Unfortunately, he was also a big head. He despised all other doctors, especially Asclepiades, but was enormously impressed by his own cleverness. Most of the information we have about him is from what he himself wrote – so it is difficult to decide how good he really was.

Biography

Galen was born in the Greek Empire in AD 129. He died in about AD 203. His family were rich. His mother sounds an interesting character. Galen tells us that she was always shouting at his father and that she used to bite her servants!

Galen also tells us that when he was a teenager Asclepios told his father in a dream to let his son study medicine. Galen studied for 12 years, and spent some of this time at the great medical school at Alexandria. In AD 157 he returned home and became a surgeon looking after gladiators for four years. The terrible wounds he had to treat taught him a lot about anatomy. But Galen was ambitious to become famous and he soon left for Rome where he spent nearly all the rest of his career.

In Rome he soon made a name for himself by his public performances – giving lectures and anatomical demonstrations. His great party trick was to cut the nerves in the neck of a pig while the pig continued to squeal. He then announced he would stop the pig squealing and he cut one of the nerves in the throat. When the pig stopped making a noise everyone was very impressed. Within a year he had become the Emperor's doctor and remained in Imperial service for the rest of his life.

Here is a story he tells about himself. His books are full of stories like this one.

Source A

A medieval illustration showing Galen experimenting on a pig.

Source B

The case of the Emperor Marcus Aurelius was quite wonderful. A messenger brought me to the Emperor. Three doctors had watched him since dawn, they had felt his pulse and thought it was the beginning of a fever. The Emperor asked me to feel his pulse. It seemed to me that his pulse, compared with the normal, was far from showing the onset of fever. My impression was that his stomach was overloaded with food, and that the food had turned into phelgm. The Emperor praised my diagnosis three times. From this time he never stopped praising me. 'He is the First of Doctors,' he said.

Galen's methods

Galen argued that first-hand observation was vital. He did this in two ways:

Diagnosing patients

Patients flocked to him for a diagnosis. He spent hours talking with patients and could sometimes diagnose just from what they told him about their lifestyle. But he also examined them carefully to find out the state of the humours. Galen's advice to doctors is given in Sources C, D, and E.

He also examined their blood, nasal passages and even their faeces.

Carrying out experiments

Galen insisted that doctors must know about the structure of the human body. Unlike Hippocrates, who did not dissect, Galen dissected apes, sheep, pigs and even an elephant's heart. He stressed the need to repeat dissections over and over again to check the results. He was a great showman and loved nothing more than giving public demonstrations of his cleverness. Here are some examples of his experiments on animals:

– to show how the nervous system worked he:

- stopped the heart beating by cutting the nerves to the heart from the brain, proving that the old idea that nerves come from the heart was wrong
- cut the nerves in the neck and showed how the shoulder was paralysed
- cut nerves in the throat to show the loss of voice.

– to show that kidneys produce urine he tied the ducts into which urine passes from the bladder to show the kidneys swelling.

His ideas on anatomy were based on studies of human skeletons (he may have dissected human corpses at Alexandria), his work with gladiators and experiments on animals. Source D shows that he realised how important using human bones was.

What he found out

Anatomy

His careful dissection of pigs and apes allowed him to discover a lot of new information about anatomy. His descriptions of bones and muscles were often accurate. However, because much of his work was based on animals, he did make mistakes. He claimed that human jaws are made from two bones like animals, when they really are made from a single bone, and he said that the right kidney is higher than the left one – this is wrong for humans but right for apes!

He found out a lot about how the nervous system works, as we have seen. He knew that the brain was important for movement and the senses. Source E is his account of an experiment on a pig.

He also developed a theory about movement of the blood which was wrong, but was a big advance at the time.

One generally obtains the major indications of fevers from the pulse, and the urine. It is essential to add to these other signs, as Hippocrates taught, such as those that appear in the face, the breathing, the presence of headache. The heart and all the arteries pulsate with the same rhythm. You could not find any arteries more convenient for taking the pulse than those in the wrists, for they are easily visible. When the pulse is hectic there will be a fever.

Source C

Human bones are subjects of study with which you should first become perfectly familiar. You cannot merely read about the bones in books, even my own book which is much more reliable than any previous book. Handle each bone so that you become a first-hand observer. At Alexandria this is very easy, since the physicians give their students opportunities for personal inspection at postmortems. If you cannot get to Alexandria it is still possible to study human bones. I have very often had the chance to do this where tombs have become broken up. Once I examined the skeleton of a robber lying on the side of the road. If you do not have the luck to see anything like this, still you can dissect an ape. Choose apes which resemble man.

Source D

Now assume that the spinal marrow lies exposed. If you wish to paralyse all parts of the body below this section then cut the spinal marrow completely through. If you cut it near the thoracic vertebrae, then the animal's breathing and voice have been damaged.

Source E

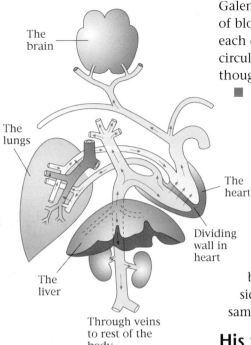

Galen understood the importance of the heart regulating the flow of blood. He knew that the veins and arteries are separate from each other. In fact he got very close to discovering that blood circulates around the body, but in the end he got it all wrong. He thought that:

■ blood was made in the liver. Some of this blood travelled through the veins to the organs of the body. It took nourishment to them and was used up.

■ other blood went through veins to the right ventricle of the heart. Some went to the lungs, some went through invisible pores in the dividing wall down the middle of the heart to the other side of the heart where it mixed with air and then through arteries to the rest of the body where it was used up.

What did Galen get wrong? Blood is not made in the liver, blood does not get used up, blood does not move from one side of the heart to the other and Galen failed to realise that the same blood circulates all the time.

His treatments – use of opposites

Galen lived 600 years after Hippocrates but he also believed in the Four Humours. In fact, he brought back into fashion Hippocrates' ideas after they had been rejected by Asclepiades. He accepted that the stomach turned food into the humours which had to be kept in balance. What he added was the idea that 'opposites' could be used to keep the humours in balance.

He was famous for encouraging blood-letting as a treatment for almost any disease. If a disease was caused by an excess of a humour then blood-letting would get rid of this excess. Hippocrates would not have approved of this amount of blood-letting because he always tried to keep treatment to a minimum and allow nature to do the healing. He was probably right because too much blood-letting could weaken patients. Galen believed in blood-letting so much that he claimed women were protected from many diseases because they menstruated. Galen also recommended other treatments based on the same idea e.g. cucumber would cool if the illness was caused by too much heat; pepper would balance a body suffering from too much cold.

Source F

A diagram of Galen's theory.

An illustration from the 15th century. It shows Galen supervising the use of an enema – liquid injected into the rectum to empty the bowel of faeces.

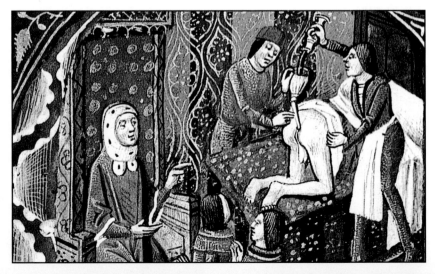

His influence

Galen was important during his lifetime because he revived Hippocratic methods, but why were his ideas believed for the next 1500 years?

- The first reason is simply that he wrote so much – over 350 books. He even employed 20 scribes to write down everything he said. And he was clever about what he wrote. Much of it was a summary of all the best bits of Hippocratic medicine. He brought it all together into one system and one body of writing. This means that it was Galen's version of Hippocrates that was handed on to later generations. He gave the impression that he was perfecting Hippocrates' work.

- By writing so much Galen gave the impression he had solved everything and so when he died nobody bothered to research into the human body any more. Galen was so famous and so confident in his own opinions that people really did think he had found all the answers.

- Living 600 years after Hippocrates, his books summarised the best of Hippocratic and other medicine, put it into a system and added his own advances. His books tell how good he was and how bad other doctors were. He often accuses other doctors of being greedy for money.

- The final reason is really down to chance. After Galen died Christianity became the official religion of the Roman Empire. Christianity gradually spread across Europe and the Church became very powerful. Galen was not a Christian but he did believe in only one god. He believed the human body had been created by this one god. A lot of his work shows how the body works together as one system. He also believed the body was ruled over by the soul. All this made Galen's ideas acceptable to the Church and later to Muslims. The idea that the human body had been perfected by God led the Church to ban any human dissection and so nobody could check Galen's ideas.

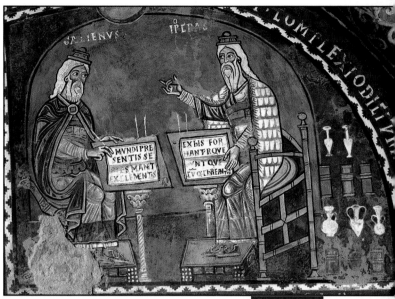

Source H

A 13th-century wall painting from a church. It shows Hippocrates with Galen.

We will leave the last word to Galen himself.

I have done as much for medicine as Trajan did for the Roman Empire when he built bridges and roads through Italy. It is I, and I alone, who have revealed the true methods of treating disease. It must be admitted that Hippocrates prepared the way, but he did not follow it up; his works have grave limitations. He marked out the road, I have made it passable.

Source I

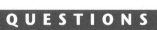

QUESTIONS

1 From the text and sources find two examples of each of the following: Galen's arrogance, his use of old ideas, his methods, his new ideas, his mistakes.

2 All the illustrations of Galen come from the Middle Ages or later. Why do you think this was?

3 What was Galen's most important contribution to medicine?

4 Explain the differences and the similarities between the ideas and methods of Hippocrates and Galen.

Public health

The Romans copied many things from the Greeks and they did not develop new ideas about the causes of disease. However their common-sense approach to medicine, and their great skills as builders and engineers did lead them to make a major contribution to medical development – public health.

They knew that large numbers of people could not live close together and be safe from disease without three things: a pure water supply, clean streets, and efficient sewers.

❶
Water was collected from rivers and springs. Vitruvius, a retired engineer in the first century BC, tells us about the trouble the Romans took only to use sources of pure water: 'You must study the soil. In clay and fine gravel, water will be poor in quality and taste; in coarse gravel it will be sweeter and purer; in lava it will be plentiful and good. If the spring is free-running and open, look at the people who use it: if they are strong, have fresh complexions and clear eyes, then the water is good.'

❷
It flowed along stone channels about the size of a doorway. The channels had stone walls, floor and roof. Sometimes these were under the ground but when valleys had to be crossed they were on bridges.

❸
When the channels got close to Rome they emerged from the hills and were carried to the city on a bridge on a long row of stone arches. The Aqua Claudia swept into the city on a bridge of over a thousand arches (it was 10 km long and 25 metres high).

❺
Once inside the city the water was piped underground to street fountains, from which most people drew their water, and to the public baths and lavatories. The rich and businesses paid a fee to have their houses and workshops connected to the system. Their connecting pipes would be limited to a certain size to make sure they didn't take too much water. Some people stole water by secretly connecting their houses to the pipes. In times of drought the public fountains, baths and lavatories had priority over private houses.
This system provided 300 gallons of water a day for every person in Rome. This is more than each of us uses today! By the fourth century AD there were 1352 public fountains and 144 public lavatories.

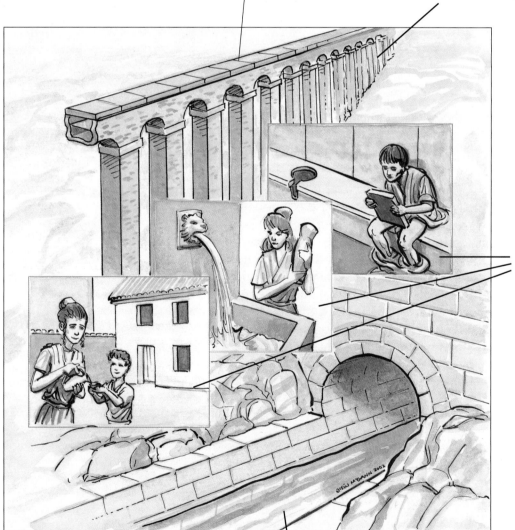

Source A

Water supply and sewage system in ancient Rome.

❹ The water was cleaned by the use of settling basins and reservoirs along the route. These allowed any dirt to sink to the bottom and leave the water pure.

The Romans did not know about germs and so they did not understand the real cause of disease. However, they used their common sense and realised that dirt, sewage, bad water and marshes were all connected to people becoming ill. The important thing is that the Romans then went and *did* something about it!

You will remember that the Greeks took great trouble to keep clean and healthy, but only the rich had the time to do this properly. You will also remember that Greek cities were described as having poor water supplies. For the Greeks, keeping clean and healthy was a private thing that each person did for themselves. For the Romans it was important that whole cities were kept clean and healthy. It was the government's job to achieve this.

The siting of towns

The starting point for the Romans was to build cities, towns, villas and army bases in healthy places. Marcus Verro mentioned this when he wrote: 'When building a house place it where it is exposed to health-giving winds. Care should be taken when there are swamps nearby because tiny creatures breed there. These float through the air and cause serious diseases.' Unfortunately Rome was built near swamps. The Romans knew that malaria came from mosquitoes and swamps and tried to drain the marshes. They were only partially successful and Rome suffered from several epidemics of malaria.

Water supply

The Romans realised that clean and pure water was important. By the end of the first century AD they had built nine aqueducts bringing water to Rome. These aqueducts were magnificent building achievements and some of them still stand today.

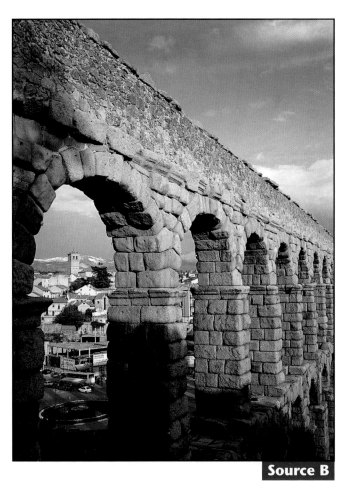

Source B

The Romans brought public health facilities to many towns in their empire. This aqueduct was built in the Spanish town of Asagovia. It is still in working order.

Compare such important engineering works carrying so much water with the idle pyramids and the useless though famous buildings of the Greeks.

Source C

Julius Frontinus, Water Commissioner for Rome, AD 97.

QUESTIONS

1 What point is Julius Frontinus making in Source C?

Public baths

The public baths were magnificent buildings and played an important part in the everyday life of Romans. People went to the baths to stay clean, as a treatment for complaints like backache, and to meet friends or even to conduct business. Some baths were huge and could take over 1,500 bathers at a time – one had over 3,000 rooms! There were warm baths, cold baths and steam baths with professional masseurs on hand. Central heating was provided by hot air circulating beneath the floor. There were also spectacular gardens with fountains and springs, and tree-lined promenades for walking. By fourth century AD Rome had 11 public baths and 856 baths in private houses.

A day at the baths

- Enter about 1pm and pay. Have a game of tennis to get warmed up.
- Enter the tepidarium, a moderately warm room, and sweat with your clothes on.
- Undress in the apodyterium and get anointed with oil. It may be mixed with African sand if you are very dirty.
- Move into the calidarium or hot room and sweat, then into the laconicum, a spot over the furnace – very hot.
- Then have water poured over you, first warm, then tepid and finally cold.
- You are then scraped with a strigil, a curved metal tool with a groove to collect all the dirt.
- Then you are sponged and re-anointed with oil.
- Finally you are plunged into the cold bath, the frigidarium.
- At last you can meet with friends, sit around the baths and chat, and later go to dinner.

A diagram showing how the rooms in the public baths were heated.

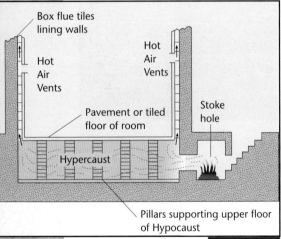

Box flue tiles lining walls

Hot Air Vents

Hot Air Vents

Pavement or tiled floor of room

Stoke hole

Hypercaust

Pillars supporting upper floor of Hypocaust

Source D

A plan of the bath house at the Roman fort Vindolanda on Hadrian's Wall in Britain. Most of it was built around AD 160 but the key shows that additions were made. A: changing room; B: cold plunge bath; C: lobby; D: warm room; E: hot, moist room; F: hot plunge bath; G: hot douche; H: uncertain; I: hot, dry room; J: stoke hole, with boiler platform and steps; K: stoke hole L:uncertain; M: latrine; N: cold douche.

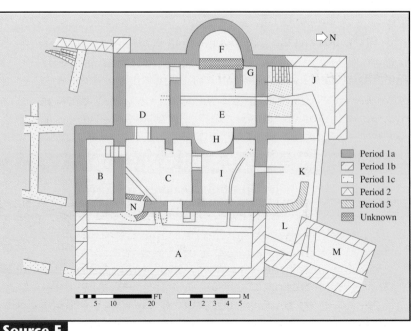

N

F

G

J

D

E

H

B

C

I

K

N

L

A

M

Period 1a
Period 1b
Period 1c
Period 2
Period 3
Unknown

FT
5   10   20

M
1 2 3 4 5

Source E

Lavatories and sewers

To keep Rome clean and healthy used water and sewage had to be got rid of. To do this the Romans built the Cloaca Maxima, a complex system of sewers and conduits running under buildings and streets and emptying into the River Tiber. Prisoners were used to clean out these sewers and they became a popular place for women to leave unwanted babies!

The sewers were connected to the public baths and lavatories, and rich families paid to have their houses connected. For those not connected to the sewers there were cesspits, or chamber pots, which could be emptied through the window into the streets below. Both the cesspits and the streets were emptied of rubbish every night and generally the streets of Rome were kept clean. Urine was useful for cleaning newly woven cloth. Fullers, keen to get their hands on as much urine as possible, would put jars outside their workshops for the public to use.

Romans might spend hours chatting with their neighbours in public lavatories like those in Source G. Under the seat was a trench with running water. In front of the seat was another trench containing running water. This was for cleaning themselves. Buckets with sponges were provided. If you think this doesn't sound very attractive, remember that London did not have public lavatories until 1851!

Other ways Rome was kept clean and healthy

- At first the city of Rome grew haphazardly with crooked, narrow streets and crowded houses. However, after a fire in AD 64 much of the city was rebuilt and the Romans took care to build straight broad streets and wide squares.

- Officials were appointed to check food being sold for quality and freshness.

- Burying the dead inside the city walls was banned and this made the much healthier method of cremation popular.

Elsewhere in the Empire

Wherever the Romans built towns, they built public baths and aqueducts. In Roman Britain most large towns like Wroxeter were supplied with pure water by aqueducts. Stone sewers were built in towns like Colchester and York, and every town would also have large public baths.

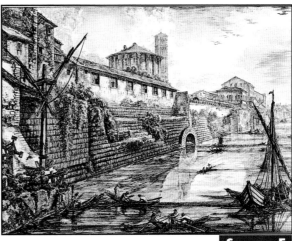

Source F

The outlet into the River Tiber of the Cloaca Maxima.

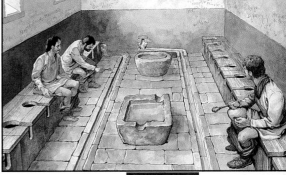

Source G

An artist's impression of Roman public lavatories.

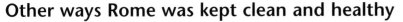

QUESTIONS

2 You have been working as the Commissioner for Public Health in Rome for a number of years. You are now planning to sell the idea of a public system to towns around the Empire. Design a four-page brochure with illustrations. Your brochure must explain (i) how the Rome public health system works, and (ii) why it is such a good system.

Why were the Romans able to provide such impressive public health facilities?

After the fall of the Roman Empire it took Europe nearly 2000 years to provide public health facilities that were anywhere near as good as those of the Romans.

The Romans concentrated on public health because:

- they realised it was important. They observed that pure water and keeping clean helped to keep disease away. They did not know why (they did not know about germs) but they knew it worked

- they had an empire to defend and it was vitally important to them to keep their people fit and healthy

- they were able to build these facilities. They were skilled engineers and builders and liked to concentrate on practical problems like the construction of a sewer rather than trying to come up with theories about the causes of disease.

The importance of the army

The army was very important to the Romans. It was the army that created and defended the Empire. The Romans, therefore, put a lot of effort into making sure the soldiers were healthy. Some of the most impressive public health achievements of the Romans can be found in remote army bases (see Source E on page 46). Many forts had bath houses and running water. The Romans did not build many hospitals – except at forts. Such hospitals were built for all army forts along the frontiers of the Empire. They were carefully planned and well stocked with instruments and medical supplies.

A few years ago, several of the original military hospitals of about 100 AD were discovered in the Rhine and Danube valleys. These were probably hospitals for frontier forces. The ground plans reveal long corridors from which opened a series of suites – each of the latter containing two private rooms connected by a small hall. In addition there were central courts for kitchens, dining rooms, pharmacies. There were no wards so each soldier patient enjoyed considerable privacy. Many surgical instruments have been found in the ruins, indicating that advanced Roman wound-surgery was used for the troops.

Source H

From a 21st-century book about the history of medicine.

QUESTIONS

3 'The Romans built a public health system partly because they needed to, and partly because they were able to.' Explain how far you agree with this statement.

The Romans were not perfect!

Because Roman public health was so impressive there is a danger in thinking that Roman cities were spotless places where no one ever caught disease. This is not true.

> We live in a city shored up with stays and props. That's how our landlords stop the buildings collapsing. They tell us we can sleep secure, when all the time the building is poised like a house of cards. There are other dangers: those cracked and leaking chamber pots people toss out through the window.

Source A

A Roman's description of living in Rome.

There are criticisms we can make of Roman public health.

- Many poor Romans lived in crowded tenement blocks. They depended on wells and water carriers for their water.

- Rome suffered from many epidemics of malaria and plague. The closely built tenement blocks helped them to spread. Between AD 164 and 189 there was a smallpox epidemic which killed 2,000 people a day at its height.

- The Romans used lead pipes for the water supply. The Romans would not have known, but this must have given lead poisoning to some people.

- The sewers of Rome emptied into the River Tiber which must have polluted the river.

- The Romans built few hospitals. The army had them, some doctors used their homes for caring for rich patients, and some big households had hospitals for their slaves. But for most of the population there were no hospitals.

This carving dates from the first century AD. It shows, very clearly, the packed buildings and narrow streets of the town of Avezzano. This shows us what Rome was probably like.

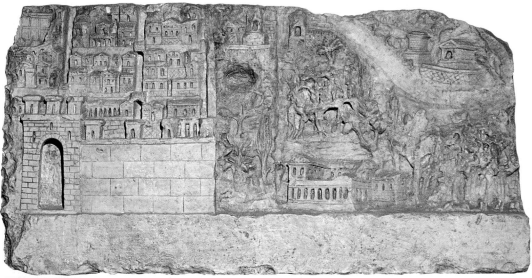

Source B

Surgery

Romans had more time for surgery than other branches of medicine. It suited their practical approach and did not involve having to come up with theories about disease.

Another reason why the Romans made advances in surgery was that it was needed to treat the wounds of Roman soldiers. As you have seen the army was very important to the Romans. One Roman writer said that war was the best school for surgeons.

Celsus wrote the most important Roman books about surgery. They contained a lot of new information:

- how to carry out plastic surgery on the nose, lips and ears

- good advice on the care of wounds: 'Let nothing be undertaken until the inside of the wound has been cleaned, lest any congealed blood remain within it. For this will turn to pus and cause inflammation which will prevent the wound from healing'

- he gave the four key signs of inflammation – redness, heat, pain, swelling. Medical students still learn these today

- treatment for broken bones e.g. what he has to say about the use of splints and bandaging is all excellent. Bleeding vessels were burnt with a cauterising iron if bleeding was not stopped by a pressure bandage

- he describes operations on wounds in the abdomen, varicose veins and cutting away scrofula, and many other operations that were not performed again until hundreds of years after the Romans.

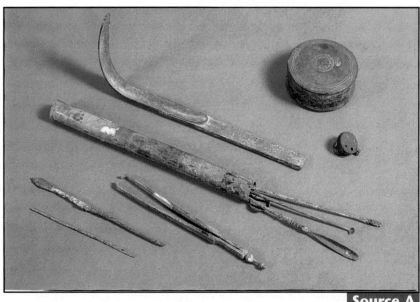

Roman surgical instruments found in a surgeon's tomb. At the top there is a medicine box and a strainer. Then a scraper (known as a strigil). An instrument case containing a probe with a threaded end for cleaning, a small spoon and a long spatula. At the bottom there are tweezers or forceps, a scalpel, and a needle.

Source A

When the doctor has carefully cut his nails and lubricated his left hand, he inserts two fingers slowly into the patient's rectum, while applying the right hand to the lower abdomen. The stone is first sought in the bladder neck and, if there, can be brought out with little trouble. If the stone has receded the fingers are pushed up towards the upper part of the bladder. The stone is brought down with caution.

An incision should then be made in the skin near the anus going to the bladder neck. This will expose the stone. If it is small it can be pulled out with the fingers. If it is bigger, a specially constructed hook must be got round it. One can then easily draw out the stone.

Celsus' description of removing a bladder stone.

Source B

QUESTIONS

1 Explain ways in which Roman surgery was more advanced than Greek surgery. Why do you think this was?

HELP YOUR REVISION

Factors

■ Galen made important advances.

■ Roman engineering skills were important for building the public health system.

■ Roman medicine developed because of the army.

Ideas about disease

■ Gods cause disease.

■ The Romans continued to believe in the Theory of the Four Humours.

Other important points

■ The Romans were very practical and made advances in public health and surgery.

■ Roman public health was not perfect.

■ They used many ideas from the Greeks.

■ Supernatural and natural approaches were used side by side (e.g. Asclepios and public health).

■ They knew there was a connection between cleanliness and health.

■ Galen brought back, and developed, Hippocrates' ideas.

EXAM PRACTICE QUESTIONS

(a) Briefly describe the main features of the Roman public health system.

(b) Explain how the Roman approach to public health was different from that of the Greeks.

(c) How far was the Roman public health system totally successful?

SOURCE INVESTIGATION

Were the Greeks more important than the Romans?

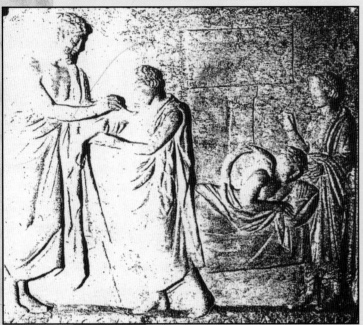

Both civilisations made contributions to the development of medicine. The popular view is that the Greeks were more interested in ideas while the Romans made more practical contributions. But who made the biggest contribution to the development of medicine, the Greeks or the Romans? Now that you know all about the Greeks and Romans you are in a position to complete this source investigation.

You probably already have some ideas of your own. Here are some to get you started.

1 The Greeks came first and the Romans did use a lot of their ideas.

2 The Greeks were the first to develop natural explanations of illness.

3 The Romans did a lot more for public health.

4 The Greeks were more interested in ideas.

5 The Romans were more practical.

Source A

A stone carving, from the fourth century BC, found in an Asclepeion. On the right the patient is being licked by a snake while he sleeps. While asleep he dreams that he is being cured by Asclepios.

The sources will give you lots of information but remember:

■ they will not cover all the points you have learnt about the Greeks and the Romans so don't be afraid to use what you know in addition to what is in the sources

■ not all the sources can be trusted: they might be biased, or just wrong.

An inscription from the second century AD found at the Asclepeion at Epidaurus.

A man with an abscess within his abdomen. When asleep in the temple of Asclepios he had a dream. It seemed to him that the god ordered the servants who accompanied him to grip him and hold him tightly so that he could cut open his abdomen. The man tried to get away, but they gripped him and bound him. Asclepios cut his belly open, removed the abscess and, after having stitched him up again, released him from his bonds. Whereupon he walked out, but the floor was covered in blood.

Source B

Q1 Study Sources A and B.
Inscriptions and carvings like these were left in Asclepeions. Does this mean that people really were cured by Asclepios? Explain your answer.

Chest trouble is announced by sweating, a salty bitter taste in the mouth, pain in the ribs and shoulder blades, trembling hands and dry coughs. The patients should be treated with a mixture of radishes, mustard and purslane pounded together and mixed with warm water. These will cause an easy and healing vomiting.

Source C

From a book by Diocles, a Greek doctor in the fourth century BC.

Q2 Study Sources B and C.
What can we learn about Greek medicine from these two sources? Explain your answer.

There is no doubt that all these doctors, in their hunt for popularity by means of some new idea, did not hesitate to buy it with our lives. Hence those quarrelsome consultations at the bedside of the patients. Hence too that gloomy inscription on monuments 'It was the crowd of doctors which killed me'.

It was not medicine that our forefathers condemned but doctors. Our forefathers refused to pay fees to profiteers in order to save their lives. Of all the Greek arts, it is only medicine which we serious Romans have not yet practised.

Source E

Q3 Study Sources D and E.
Does Source E prove that Source D is wrong? Explain your answer.

During a severe plague in Rome in 293 BC, the advice obtained was to ask for help from the Greek god Asclepios, at his temple in Epidaurus. The Romans were directed by the priests of Epidaurus to build a similar temple in Rome, and were presented with a sacred serpent. Accordingly a temple was built on an island of the River Tiber.

Source D

From a 20th-century book about the Romans.

Pliny, a Roman, writing in the first century AD.

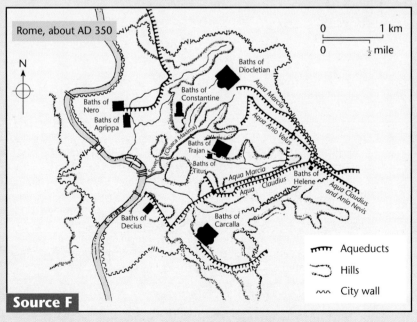

Source F

A map of Rome in about 350 AD. The blue river is the River Tiber.

Q4 Study Source F.
What does this source tell you about Roman attitudes towards medicine? Explain your answer.

SOURCE INVESTIGATION

Just when the lamps were lit, a messenger came and brought me to the Emperor. Three doctors had watched over him since dawn, and two of them felt his pulse, and all three thought a fever attack was coming. The Emperor asked me to feel his pulse. My impression was that the pulse was far from indicating a fever attack, but that his stomach was stuffed with food he had eaten. The Emperor praised my diagnosis and said 'That is it. It is just as you say. I have eaten too much cold food.'

It is I, and I alone, who has revealed the true path of medicine. It must be admitted that Hippocrates already staked out this path. He prepared the way, but I have made it passable.

Source G

Galen describing his work for the Roman Emperor, Marcus Aurelius, in the second century AD.

Q5 Study Source G.
Do you think that Source G is reliable? Explain your answer.

When the gangrene has developed, the limb must be amputated. Between the healthy and the diseased part, the flesh is cut through with a scalpel down to the bone actually over a joint, and it is better that some of the sound part should be cut away than any diseased part should be left behind. The bone is then to be cut through with a small saw.

Source H

From a medical encyclopaedia written by a Roman in the first century AD.

Q6 Study Sources H and I.
Are you surprised that both these sources come from Roman times? Explain your answer.

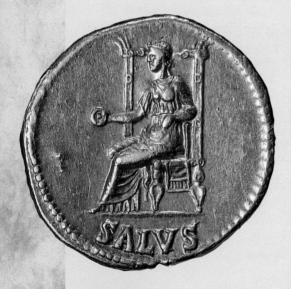

Source I

An engraving on a Roman coin. It shows Salus, the Roman goddess of health. She was the Roman equivalent of the Greek goddess Hygeia.

In 292 BC Asclepios was brought to Rome at a time of emergency. The first Greek doctor to settle in Rome was the wound specialist Archagathus who came in 219 BC. At first he was highly regarded and given citizenship; but as a result of his savage use of the knife he was nicknamed 'executioner' and all doctors became hated.

In 46 BC Julius Caesar gave citizenship to all who practised medicine in Rome and by the first century AD Greek medicine was almost totally dominant in Rome. Important Roman contributions to medicine were more practical – for example, improvements in public health engineering and the invention of the military hospital.

Source J

From a book about the history of medicine published in 1997.

Q7 Study all the sources.
'The Romans were less important than the Greeks in the development of medicine.' How far do the sources support this statement?

25

How much do you know?

It is now time to see if we can bring together what we have covered so far. We are looking for developments and patterns. You need to copy these charts on to a sheet of A3 paper and then complete them.

Find examples for:

	Prehistoric	Egyptian	Greek	Roman
Ideas about causes of illness – supernatural				
Ideas about causes of disease – natural		e.g. blocking of the body's channels		
Treatments – supernatural				
Treatments – natural				
Trained doctors?				
Code of conduct for doctors?				
Surgery				
Public health				
Important individuals				

As you go through this book you are going to find examples of factors like war and religion helping and hindering progress in medicine. You can keep a list of these examples at the back of your exercise book or folder. These will be very helpful when you need to revise for examinations.

	Helping	Hindering
War	e.g. Galen and gladiators	
Religion		
Government		
Individuals		
Philosophy and Science		

Did nothing change in the Middle Ages?

For the exam you will need to know:

☑ Whether the Christian Church helped or hindered the development of medicine

☑ Whether many ideas from the Greeks and Romans were still used

☑ How much change there was between the beginning and the end of the Middle Ages

☑ Whether Islamic medicine was more advanced than European medicine.

The problem of the Middle Ages!

We use the term 'The Middle Ages' to describe the period between the fall of Rome in 476 and the Renaissance which started in the 1400s.

Here are some judgements by historians about medicine in the Middle Ages.

A thousand years of darkness.

Galen was the final star that shone and when he died there settled over Europe a darkness that was not lifted for many centuries.

The rational medicine of the Greeks and the Romans descends into darkness.

However, there are some problems with these judgements, and even with the idea of the Middle Ages!

The fall of the Roman Empire

Two important developments dominate the beginning of the Middle Ages:

■ the fall of the Roman Empire

■ the rise of Christianity.

The Roman Empire took hundreds of years to collapse. By the fourth century it was under pressure from large numbers of Goths. In 364 it split into two halves and by the end of the sixth century the Western Empire had disintegrated into kingdoms ruled by the invading Goths, Huns and Vandals. In the ninth century there was another round of invasions, this time by the Vikings from Scandinavia. The great cities of the Roman Empire had fallen into ruin. All of this meant that many of the achievements from earlier times were lost e.g. public health systems and medical libraries. In many areas there was a return to a combination of folk medicine, supernatural approaches, and practical common-sense remedies. It was not until the 12th century that some kind of peace and stability returned to Europe.

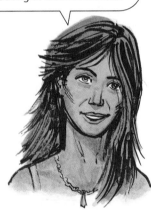

The term 'the Middle Ages' really only applies when we look at developments in Europe. You will see that it does not mean much when we are looking at Islamic medicine.

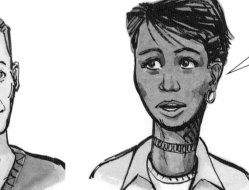

It was not one continuous period. For example, some historians call the first 600 years immediately after the fall of the Roman Empire 'The Dark Ages' because this was when there was a lot of fighting and destruction. Later in the Middle Ages things became more peaceful and settled.

The usual idea people have of the Middle Ages is that everything went downhill after the fall of the Roman Empire and there was no progress until the Renaissance came along. Is this true?

Christianity

After the death of Christ, Christianity grew from being an insignificant movement in the Roman province of Palestine to become the major religion of Europe. At first, Roman Emperors persecuted Christians. This all changed in the fourth century when the Emperor Constantine was converted to Christianity. In 313 he made it one of the official religions of the Empire and by the fifth century it was the only official religion.

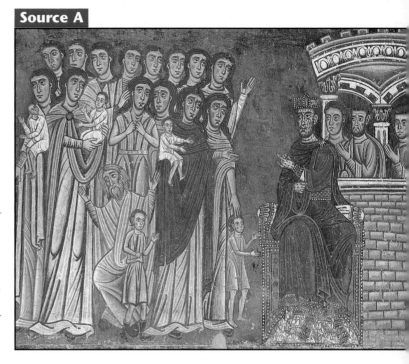

Source A

In this 13th-century illustration the Emperor Constantine is shown suffering from leprosy. He is rejecting pagan advice to cure it by bathing in the blood of 3,000 children (their mothers are appealing to him). Instead, he calls for a Christian saint, is cured, and is converted to Christianity.

Christianity had an enormous impact on medicine – but was this impact good or bad?

Christianity did not encourage people to be worried about physical illness.	However, there were also reasons why Christians should take an interest in healing.

Christians thought the soul was more important than the body. Their main concern was to save people's souls.

↓

Disease was thought to be a punishment from God for sins committed. If this was so, then it was right for the person who was ill to suffer. Cures should only come from God.

Christians had believed that Christ's Second Coming was near. This would be the 'Day of Judgement' and the ending of this life on earth. This made earthly problems seem unimportant.

As time went by and the Second Coming did not happen, Christians began to take more interest in medicine. After all, they could not simply ignore the fact that people were ill!

↓

In the Gospels there are many examples of Jesus healing people. This led to Christians arguing that they had a duty to follow Jesus' example and show compassion for fellow humans by caring for the sick. However, it would still be God providing the cure, through those who were providing care.

↓

Many monasteries cared for the sick. The Benedictine monks believed that 'the care of the sick is to be placed above and before every other duty'

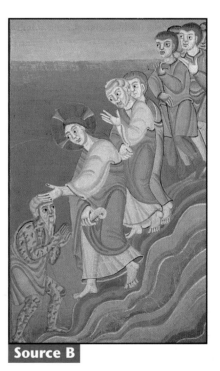

Source B

This 11th-century illustration shows Jesus healing a leper.

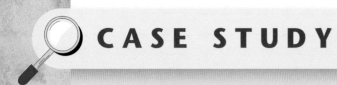

CASE STUDY

Anglo-Saxon Medicine – The Dark Ages?

To find out what medicine was like at the beginning of the Middle Ages we are going to use Anglo-Saxon medicine as a case study. The Angles and the Saxons were German tribes who began invading, and settling, in England in the fifth century – the so-called Dark Ages.

Most of the evidence we have about medicine in Anglo-Saxon times comes from skeletons and artefacts, and from Leech books (these contained details of illnesses and treatments. Doctors were called Leeches).

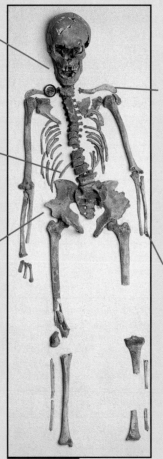

many of her teeth were destroyed by decay (caused by too much ale and honey) and when she died she only had the infected roots left and abscesses – very painful

her left collar bone has been fractured but it was set and healed well

she had arthritis in her lower back and backbone – painful and made everyday actions like carrying and bending difficult

she was born with a deformed pelvis

she wore a bronze bracelet on her left wrist

The skeleton of a woman who was buried in the fifth century. She died in her thirties and was 157 cm (5ft 2 in) tall.

Source A

The contents of other grave sites show:

- ■ short life expectancy
- ■ high infant mortality
- ■ women dying young, particularly in childbirth
- ■ a lot of bone and joint diseases like rheumatism and arthritis.

If we look at how they lived, none of this is surprising.

Their housing was primitive with most people living in small, damp, dark hovels – one dirty and draughty room heated by a fire. Sanitation was primitive and dysentery was common.

Their diet largely consisted of wheat and barley, bread, beans and peas. They seem to have had little red meat – so were short of crucial vitamins, especially Vitamin C. This lowered resistance to disease.

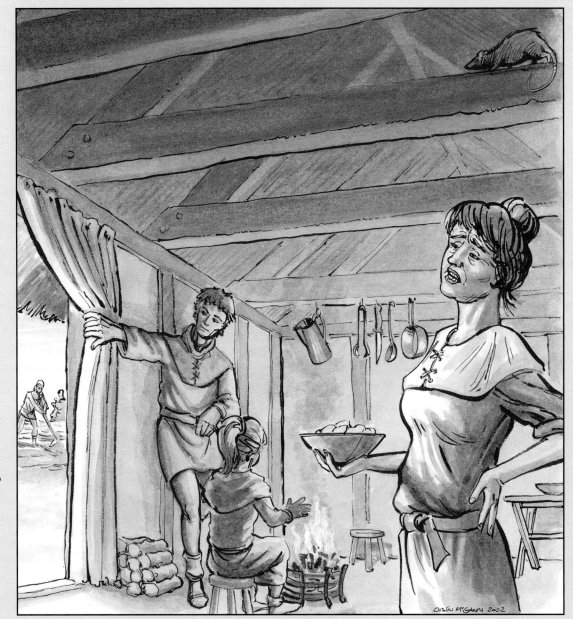

Their working conditions did not help – long hours of labour in the fields. They were poorly clothed, and were constantly damp and wet leading to rheumatism and arthritis.

They caught many diseases from parasites from animals like sheep – leading to vomiting and diarrhoea. Malaria was common, as were eye infections and skin diseases.

Q1 You have to write a report about the woman in Source A. Describe her injuries and explain how her lifestyle led to these injuries.

Q2 Compare the health and lifestyle of Anglo-Saxons with those of prehistoric farmers.

Going to the doctor – Anglo-Saxon style

What would happen to you if you went to a doctor in Anglo-Saxon times? He would probably be a monk but there were some doctors outside monasteries. They were not given a formal training so they used their experience and their Leech books. The treatments given below all come from Leech books.

Cynefrith has awful tooth decay – in fact he has hardly any teeth left! In those days they thought tooth decay was caused by worms!

Werburh has a pain in her head, as well as bad toothache.

For tooth worms, take oat meal and henbane seed and wax, equal amounts of all, mix together, make into a wax candle and burn it, let it smoke into the mouth, put a black sheet under, then the worms will fall out.

From which places should blood be drawn? From 23: e.g. for complaints of the head, from two arteries at the back of the head down to the bone four finger breadths from the ear, for toothache from two arteries on the little finger of the left hand if the teeth on the right side ache.

Dun has chicken-pox.

For elfsickness [probably chicken-pox, although they thought the spots were caused by arrows fired by elves] take fennel, lupin and lichen from a holy crucifix, put a handful of each, tie up all the herbs in a cloth, dip in holy font water three times, lay the herbs on hot coals, then write a Christ's cross on every limb, and take a little handful of consecrated herbs and boil in milk, drip holy water on them three times and let him sup them before his meal.

William has already been to the doctor. He was bled but too much blood was taken and he is now feeling worse than ever!

A person weak because too much blood has been bled – If it is wintertime, we bathe the face and soles of the feet with warm water. If it is summer, we bathe the face and soles with cold water, or induce vomiting and apply odours like mustard or mint to the nostrils.

Medicine for the dimness of the eyes; take the juice of celandine, mix with bumblebees' honey, put in a brass vessel, make lukewarm over warm coals until it is cooked. [You should remember that honey kills bacteria – we have come across this before. It would help cure infection of the eyes.]

Cuthbert's eyes have been hurting him and his eyesight is being affected.

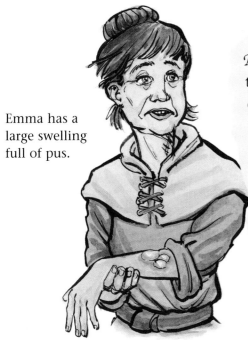

Emma has a large swelling full of pus.

Abscess of the liver. If the swelling and the pus rise so that it can be lanced and let out, prepare her by an ointment of dove's dung, and bathe the place with water and herbs. When you consider the swelling is becoming soft, touch her with the iron lancet and cut a little bit so the blood can come out. Do not release too much blood lest she becomes exhausted. When you pierce the swelling have linen bandage ready so you may bind the wound up at once, and when you want to let out more, remove the bandage. This lets it out little by little until it dries up. Clean it every day. If it should have dirty discharges, clean it with honey and draw it together again.

Athelstan suffers from worms!

If there are worms in one's insides boil green rue [a shrub] in butter, drink a cupful after a night's fast; they will go away with the stool and he will be well again.

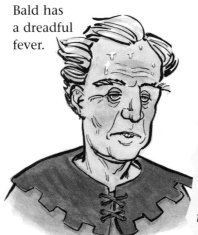

Bald has a dreadful fever.

For fever: One shall take seven little wafers such as are offered in Church, and write these names on each wafer [e.g. Constantinus]. Then one shall sing the charm first in the left ear, then in the right ear, then over the top of the man's head; and then let a virgin go up to him and hang it on his neck, and let this be done for three days.

Aldhelm has broken his leg

Bathe the broken limb and apply soothing ointment. [There is little evidence of splints being used – this means there was little chance of broken limbs healing straight and strong.]

Oxa has a pain in the jaw.

Take the spindle with which a woman spins, bind around his neck with a woollen thread and make him drink hot goat's milk; he will soon be well [hot milk was recommended by the Romans as a gargle for a sore throat].

QUESTIONS

1 Draw a chart with the following headings written across the top: magic, Christian, Greek and Romans, natural.
Down the left-hand side of the chart write the name of each patient.
Put a tick against each patient's name in the column that best describes the treatment the patient received. You can tick more than one column for each patient.

Although the Anglo-Saxons had no idea what was causing disease many of the medicines they used were natural treatments and did help patients to recover. Some of these were copied from the Romans and some they developed themselves through long and careful observation. Some of the plants, minerals and substances taken from animals that would have worked, and which are still used today in medicines, include:

- onions and garlic. These are antibiotics and kill bacteria
- copper salts, formed from the copper in brass vessels. These were scraped out and made excellent ointment for infected eyelids
- lichen. This was used for wounds and animal bites. It kills bacteria.

Treatments like these were effective and it was no accident that the Anglo-Saxon doctors used them. They knew they worked, even if they did not know why.

However, there were obvious limitations to Anglo-Saxon medicine:

- they had no anaesthetics except for some herbs like mandrake, henbane and poppy. These might have dulled pain a little – but not much. As we have already seen, they would have suffered terribly from toothache
- they seem to have used blood-letting and vomiting a lot to remove harmful humours. This would have done little good, and some harm
- magic was an important part of Anglo-Saxon medicine. It was often used alongside natural treatment
- they could do little surgery (apart from blood-letting). They also lacked antiseptics.

QUESTIONS

2 Read these two statements about Anglo-Saxon medicine. Write an essay explaining which one you agree with the most.

'Anglo-Saxon society was at the mercy of disease on the one hand, and medical ignorance, on the other. Apart from basic herbal mixtures, they had no means of treating serious illness.'

'The Anglo-Saxons took from the Greeks and Romans some of the best they had to offer and integrated it into their own treatments. Many treatments gave some comfort to the patients, and a few were positively useful. These must have been based on careful observation of patients and evaluation of the medicines. But there were illnesses for which the only resort was charms and amulets.'

Medieval hospitals – cesspools of infection?

Today we take hospitals for granted. But they have not always been important. In the Middle Ages most people would never have set foot inside one. Being born, dying, and medical care mostly took place at home.

The usual picture of medieval hospitals is one of 'gateways to death' and 'cesspools of infection'. They are meant to have been such terrible places that you were more likely to die if you went in, than if you stayed out. Let's see if this is true.

It is fair to say that without Christianity medieval hospitals would not have existed. As early as the fourth century Christians were setting up hospitals for the diseased and the needy. They were trying to carry out the teachings of Jesus – to help the sick and the poor.

Later in the Middle Ages, hospitals became larger and more impressive. In the early days most had just a few beds. By 1287 St Leonard's in York was looking after 225 patients. Hospitals in cities like Milan and Paris were even larger.

What was a hospital?

The answer to this is complicated. The word hospital was used to describe a range of different types of places.

Leper houses

Most people feared lepers. They were also disgusted by them. This was because of the physical symptoms of the disease – parts of the body are slowly eaten away leading to scaly and decaying flesh, and mutilated fingers and toes. As a result lepers were horribly deformed. Leprosy was seen as a living death for which there was no cure. Lepers were not allowed to marry, they had to dress in special clothes and ring a warning bell as they approached. Many people believed lepers were being punished by God for their sins. They also thought that leprosy was spread by sexual intercourse!

Leper houses were built on main roads on the outskirts of towns. Their main job was to keep the lepers separated from the rest of the population. They provided lodging and food, but not treatment.

By 1225 there were 19,000 leper hospitals in Europe. By 1600 they had nearly all disappeared as leprosy died out in Europe.

Almshouses

These were often very small, sometimes with just a priest and perhaps 12 inmates. These might be people too weak to look after themselves, the elderly needing long-term care, widows with young children or single pregnant women. Almshouses also gave shelter to travellers, especially pilgrims visiting holy shrines. The poor would be given a few nights' shelter, especially in winter. Although some of the people looked after would be sick, no real medical treatment was given.

> No leper shall come within the gates of the borough and if one gets in by chance, the serjeant shall put him out at once. If one wilfully forces his way in, his clothes shall be taken off him and burnt and he shall be turned out naked.

Source A

From the local laws of Berwick-upon-Tweed.

> I forbid you ever to enter churches, or go into a market, or a bakehouse, or any assemblies of people
> I forbid you ever to wash your hands or even any of your belongings in spring or stream water
> I forbid you to go out without your leper's dress
> I forbid you to have intercourse with any woman except your wife
> I forbid you to touch infants or young folk

Source B

From a 13th-century set of rules for lepers.

Hospitals

There were other places that did tend to concentrate on looking after the sick. We shall call these hospitals, but it should be remembered that they also took in people because they were poor as well as because they were sick. They varied in size enormously. Some, in big cities, had hundreds of beds, but the average was probably between 20 and 50. However, all over the countryside there were small hospitals with room for only five or six.

These hospitals were very different from today's hospitals – people who were seriously ill and needed a lot of care were often not allowed in! This was because they would take so much looking after that it would stop people from concentrating on the main purpose of the hospital which was to pray and attend services.

Source C

A map of medieval Norwich showing leper houses, almshouses and hospitals for the sick.

So, who would you find in these hospitals? – the elderly, poor widows with young children, orphans, the blind, cripples and the poor who were sick. The elderly might stay for years until they died, others might stay for a couple of weeks until they were feeling a bit better. The hungry just stayed overnight. Some hospitals concentrated on looking after certain types of people. St Bartholomew's in London looked after destitute women who were pregnant. It also supported and educated any infants of mothers who died in childbirth.

Why were hospitals built?

Most of these hospitals were built and paid for by the Church. In the 13th century 160 new hospitals were built. Walter Suffield, the Bishop of Norwich, had a hospital built during this time. He did this to try to cleanse himself of his sins and to help him get to heaven after he died. But he also saw it as his Christian duty to help the sick, the homeless and the poor. In fast-growing cities like Norwich there were many poor and homeless people – and the cold, the damp, the filth and a poor diet lacking in vitamins soon made them sick. Sickness led to worse poverty – the death of the breadwinner in a family could leave the family destitute.

QUESTIONS

1 Describe medieval attitudes towards lepers.

Another reason for helping the poor was that by getting them into these hospitals they could be won over to Christianity, and taught to live a Christian life. Many of the people who looked after the inmates were priests, monks or nuns. But many ordinary women also did much of the nursing, the cleaning and the cooking.

What was the treatment like?

Hospitals were houses of religion – during the Middle Ages they were called Houses of God rather than hospitals. Their main job was not to care for patients physically but to look after them spiritually. The inmates spent much of their day praying and confessing – they attended seven services a day. It was believed that they were poor and sick because they had sinned. They now had to be helped to rid themselves of their sins – this would help them get to heaven. They also had to say prayers for people who had donated money to the hospital. The more prayers that were said for you, the quicker you got to heaven.

It was also believed that paintings, statues, and relics of Christ, the Virgin Mary or the saints had the power to cure people.

We know little about the medical care in these hospitals. This is because it was not their main task. Some of the larger hospitals did have doctors and surgeons visiting their patients. But usually visiting doctors were only for the staff – the priests, nuns or monks who were ill. In some hospitals the monks themselves were able to carry out some basic treatment but the most important treatments patients received were: regular meals, rest, clean linen, baths, warmth and shelter. These paupers were probably better off than the rich people who were looked after in their own homes and were made weaker and weaker by purgings and blood-letting.

The work is hard. Quite often day must become night and night day, so the sick poor can be cleaned, washed, put to bed, bathed, dried, fed, given drinks, carried from one bed to another, lifted so beds can be remade, personal linen washed out every day in clean water. Every week between eight and nine hundred sheets can be rinsed in clean water, put into the wash tub, and washed in the River Seine, whether it is freezing, windy or raining, and then hung out to dry in the summer, or dried by a great fire in the winter.

Source D

A description of the work to be done in the Hôtel Dieu in Paris.

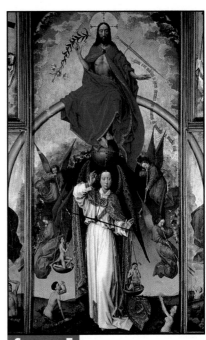

Source E

A painting, from a medieval hospital, of the Last Judgement. It shows St Michael weighing souls in the balance. The heavier has failed to carry out Christ's teachings and will descend into hell. The patients would see this painting all the time! It was to encourage people to donate money to the poor, and to encourage the poor to pray for those who had donated money.

QUESTIONS

2 Write out the following three headings:

Asclepion   Medieval hospitals   Hospitals today

For each one, list examples of the following areas: purpose, types of treatment, who paid for it, who went there. Then explain which two of the three have the most in common.

The Church and dissection

Many books about the history of medicine tell you that the Church banned human dissection in the Middle Ages. This is wrong. In 1299 the Pope banned dissected corpses from being buried in mass graves. He wanted them to have a proper Christian burial. While in 1482 a later Pope said that the Church had no objection to human dissection as long as the body came from an executed criminal.

Human dissections had begun by the end of the 13th century and were soon being used in some universities to teach students about the body. However, they did not lead to more knowledge about the human body. There were several reasons for this:

- although the Church did not ban dissections, it was not keen on them. This was because it did not like the tampering with human remains that went on e.g. people used to dig up bodies so they could move them to have them buried in a special place, other people tried to preserve the heart of the dead person

- the idea that dissections could be used to check or correct what Galen said about the body never crossed anyone's mind. Instead, they were used to illustrate Galen's ideas about the body

- frequently it was not possible to find human corpses and animals were often used – usually pigs

- some teachers did not think dissections were worth the trouble when you could find all the answers in Galen's books

- dissections could only take place in winter and had to be completed very quickly – for obvious reasons! (Think about the smell if they hung around for too long in warm weather.)

Source A

A 15th-century illustration showing the teacher reading from Galen's book while assistants dissect the corpse as students watch.

Medieval beliefs and treatments – supernatural or natural?

Christian beliefs

It is impossible for us to really understand the shock and horror caused by disease in the Middle Ages. Death came unannounced, again and again. The plague, typhus and measles regularly came and went, killing thousands. Many women died as a result of childbirth, and infant mortality was very high. Average life expectancy was about 29!

What made all this more terrifying was the belief that disease was a punishment by God for sins. It followed from this that only God could cure people of illness. This meant that cures were beyond human control.

The power of prayer

But people did what they could to try to persuade God to be merciful. They turned to prayer, and to paintings, statues and relics of Christ, the Virgin Mary and the saints. They believed these had the power of God and could cure patients. Healing shrines flourished where relics and images were collected. People flocked to Canterbury in their thousands because Becket's blood could cure blindness, leprosy and deafness! There was also the belief that as kings were appointed by God, they had supernatural healing powers. People queued to be touched by the king to be cured of scrofula (tuberculosis of a gland in the neck).

Prayer, the laying on of hands, amulets with Christian engravings, holy oil, and relics of the saints were all used. Each part of the body and each disease had its own saint – St Roch for plague, St Margaret for women in labour and so on. Many people carried passages from the Bible to fend off disease. Expectant mothers had a prayer on a piece of parchment, which was the same length as the height of Christ, wrapped round them when they gave birth.

They also believed in demons! God could tell devils to enter the body and send people mad. Those who believed that devils had entered their bodies often tried to flog or starve them out.

The Four Humours

What is difficult for us to understand is that they also believed in the Theory of the Four Humours. However, they saw nothing strange in seeking religious and natural cures alongside each other. They thought that a particular illness could often be explained by an imbalance in the humours which they could do something about, but in the long run they knew they would always be visited by disease as a punishment by God.

> If the many-footed worm, which rolls up into a ball when you touch it, is pricked with a needle, and the aching tooth is then touched with the needle, the pain will end.
> The beak of a magpie hung from the neck cures pain in the teeth.

Source B

A charm for curing toothache by John Gaddesden, an English doctor in the 14th century.

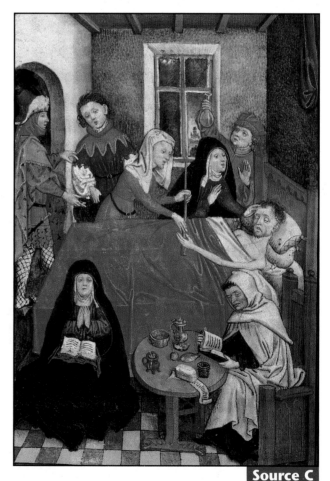

Source C

A 15th-century deathbed scene. The prayers and the last rites would help the patient get to heaven. It shows religious and natural approaches side by side, but which is more important?

Astrology

In the 14th century the use of astrology became important in medicine. There were two reasons for this:

■ more Greek books were being translated. From these people learned that Hippocrates had written that doctors should study 'the progress of the seasons and the dates of rising and setting of stars' so they could forecast changes in the weather. These changes would affect the humours in the body so doctors would be able to diagnose and treat patients better

■ scientists had begun to investigate the sky and the planets. Doctors began to accept that the planets and the signs of the zodiac had an important impact on health and illness. This made sense because the human body was made of the same basic elements as the planets.

They also believed there was a link between the signs of the zodiac and certain parts of the body e.g. Aries ruled the head. This made it important for doctors to know the position of the planets when diagnosing illnesses and deciding on a treatment. For this they had a book called a Vademecum. This told them which treatments could be used on certain parts of the body at that time. When the moon was in a particular sign it was very dangerous to treat the part of the body linked to that sign. Doctors also had to consider the position of the planets when a patient was born!

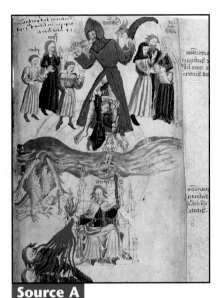

Source A

A 15th-century illustration showing how the coming together of Saturn and Jupiter in 1345 was responsible for the plague three years later. It shows Saturn at the top, eating his children, and Jupiter at the bottom casting thunderbolts.

Aries   Avoid cuts in the head and face and cut no vein in the head.

Taurus   Avoid cuts in the neck and throat and cut no veins there.

Leo   Avoid cutting the nerves, and cuts in the sides and the bones. Do not bleed the back.

Virgo   Avoid opening a wound in the belly and in internal parts.

Scorpio   Avoid cutting the testicles and anus.

Sagittarius   Avoid incisions in the thighs and fingers. Do not cut blemishes or growths.

Capricorn   Avoid cutting the knees or the veins and sinews in these places.

Gemini   Avoid cuts in the shoulders and arms or hands and cut no vein.

Cancer   Avoid cuts in the breast and sides, stomach and lungs, and cut no vein that goes to the spleen.

Libra   Avoid opening wounds in the umbilicus and parts of the belly and do not open a vein in the back or do cupping.

Aquarius   Avoid cutting the legs and places as far as the heels.

Pisces   Avoid cutting the feet.

Source B

A Zodiac man from a 14th-century Vademecum.

Galen – again!

Remember Galen? In the Middle Ages he was more important than ever! When the Roman Empire fell much of his writing was lost to Europe, although some monasteries did manage to keep and copy some of his books. Muslim doctors in the Arab world continued to study his books and produce new translations. In the 12th century contacts between the Muslim world and Europe developed and Galen's works again became widespread. One example of this is a medicine book written in the 13th century that had in it over 600 references to Galen!

After 1100 medical schools were set up and students simply learnt what was in Galen's books – nobody dared question them. This was because Galen's ideas fitted in with Christianity very easily. They suggested that every person is a microcosm of the universe, worked in the same way as the universe, and was made of the same elements (see Source E). This matched the Christian idea of God creating everything. The Church therefore gave its support to Galen's ideas – he was called 'God's servant'. Dissections were used to show students what Galen had said about the body. They were not used to test Galen's ideas and learn more. As a result, little progress was made. This was partly Galen's fault. He claimed to give all the answers to all medical questions and this was not questioned until the 16th century.

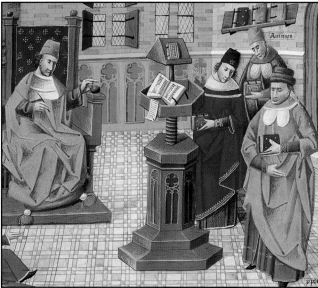

Source C

A professor at a university around 1300 showing his class the greats – Hippocrates, Galen and Avicenna.

Rise early in the morning, and straight remember,
With water cold to wash your hands and eyes,
Both comb your head and rub your teeth.

Great suppers do the stomach much offend,
Sup light if quiet you to sleep intend.
To keep good diet, you should never feed
Until you find your stomach clean and void.

Yet for your lodging rooms give this direction,
In houses where you mind to make your dwelling,
That there be no ill smells
Of puddle-waters, or of excrements.
Against humours overflowing,
Purge, vomit and let blood,
Each bad infection is withstood.

Three special Months (September, April, May)
There are, in which 'tis good to open a vein.

Source D

The rules, from the 15th century, at the medical school at Salerno, in Italy.

The Universe	Human Beings
Made up of four basic elements	Made up of four humours that match the elements
Fire (hot and dry)	yellow bile
Water (cold and wet)	phlegm or mucus
Earth (cold and dry)	black bile
Air (hot and dry)	blood

Source E

Galen's ideas on the universe and humans.

The Four Humours

At the centre of Galen's ideas were the Four Humours. These dominated medicine in the Middle Ages. Good health was achieved by keeping the humours in balance. Age, diet, the weather and lifestyle could all upset this balance. Medieval writers added their own ideas to this theory. They decided that each organ in the body had its own complexion, for example the brain was cold and moist. The body naturally rid itself of excessive humours through sweat, urine and faeces. When this was not enough, illness occurred and treatment was needed.

This diagram shows how the Theory of the Four Humours was developed and added to from Hippocratic times, through Galen and the Middle Ages. You can see that in the Middle Ages they thought the humours were affected by the signs of the zodiac.
Starting at 1 o' clock:

Crab	= Cancer
Twins	= Gemini
Bull	= Taurus
Ram	= Aries
Fishes	= Pisces
Water-carrier	= Aquarius
Goat	= Capricorn
Archer	= Sagittarius
Scorpion	= Scorpio
Balance	= Libra
Virgin	= Virgo
Lion	= Leo

Source F

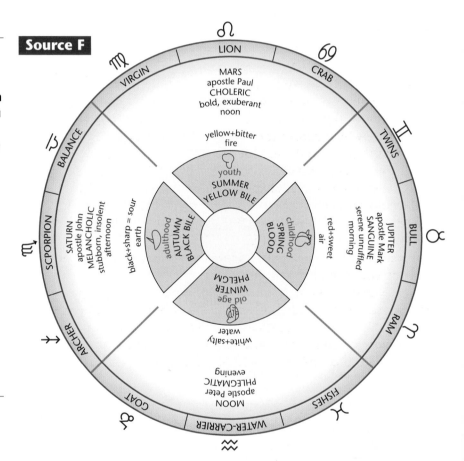

QUESTIONS

1 Did people in the Middle Ages just copy Greek ideas, or did they develop them?

2 'Medieval medicine was a mixture of supernatural and natural ideas.' How far do you agree with this statement?

Visiting a medieval doctor

As you are studying this section make notes about differences and similarities between the methods of a Greek doctor and an Anglo-Saxon doctor.

Being examined by the doctor

The first thing you would notice is that the doctor would probably not examine you! Examination of your urine was the main way of diagnosing what was wrong with patients. Its colour would show if there was too much of a particular humour in the body. The doctor would use a book showing the different colours of urine. The colour would tell him what the illness was, which part of the body was affected, and what the remedy was. He might also examine your blood and faeces, and would certainly use an astrological chart. Sometimes you might be examined, but if

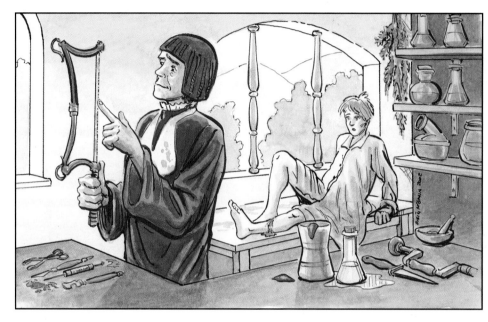

you were a woman you would remain fully clothed and would describe your symptoms to the doctor.

Sometimes the patient's pulse was taken and there might even be a physical examination. Everything that was found could be explained by the Four Humours e.g. a hard and dark lump on the body would be caused by black bile, a red swelling by too much blood. Internal complaints could be blamed on blockages in the body.

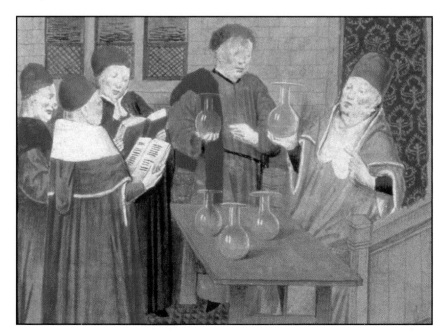

15th-century doctors examining urine samples.

Source A

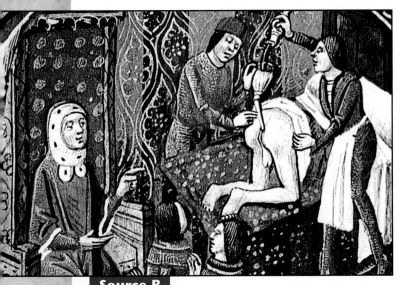

Source B

This 15th-century illustration shows Galen watching over the use of an enema.

Treatments

The aim of all treatments was to get the humours back into balance.

Medicine

You might be given medicine. All medicines were divided into four types:

- warming
- cooling
- moistening
- drying.

The right type would be chosen to get the humours back into balance. Some were used as ointments (based on wax or grease); some were swallowed (based on oil or wine).

A usual treatment was first to be given a medicine to cool your temperature a little. Ointments would then be put on the part of the body in pain either to heat or cool the humours. This would help soothe your aches and pains a little.

The medicine you might be given to swallow would be mixtures of plants, animals, or minerals. Some plants were common like clover, knapweed and dock, and could be found in the hedgerows. Others like sugar (which was used a lot), ginger, cloves and nutmeg were imported from countries like India, Persia and Egypt. Elephants' tusks, bezoar (a stone from the stomach of a goat in Persia), and powdered horns of the mythical unicorn were meant to have magical powers as was the plant verbena, which could cure the bite of a rabid dog, reduce fever, restore a nursing mother's milk, stop bleeding and keep away the plague!

Purging

If you were unlucky the doctor might try purging by vomiting or defecation – to get rid of unwanted humours. This could do you a lot of harm! You might first be given linseed fried in hot fat. If this did not work you would be given an enema (a mixture of water, wheat bran, salt, honey and herbs and soap), which was squirted into the anus through a greased pipe attached to a pig's bladder.

Bleeding

The doctor was more likely to try blood-letting. This was used to cure those already ill and to prevent healthy people becoming ill. There was so much demand for blood-letting that people with no medical training set themselves up as blood-letters.

> They gather by the hundreds at the house of the blood–letter. After he draws their blood he tells them, in order to obtain an additional fee, that he sees by their blood that they will need another blood-letting. And the fools return.

Source C

A medieval doctor comments on blood-letting.

Doctors did realise that too much bleeding was a danger. But they thought this was because it had put the humours out of balance or it had been done at the wrong time according to the Zodiac chart. But sometimes they accidentally opened an artery and the patient bled to death. Remember that they still accepted Galen's idea that the body constantly made new blood as it was used up. This meant they did not realise you would grow weak if you were bled too much!

You would probably be bled from the arm or the leg. Just below the elbow was a popular place because this would cleanse the blood and prevent illness.

If you were old or weak you were more likely to have leeches attached to your skin. These were taken from clean streams, stored for a day with no nourishment, and then applied to open wounds and swellings.

Women and children were usually cupped – a heated glass or a brass vessel was placed on the skin which had been scratched with a knife.

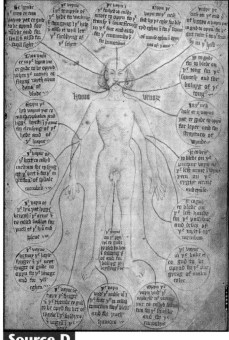

Source D

A vein man from a book belonging to a barber-surgeon (a person who carried out easy surgical procedures as well as shaving and hairdressing). It shows which parts of the body to bleed for specific illnesses e.g. bleeding from the vein between the finger and the thumb helps migraine, blood-letting from the vein under the ankle helps diseases of the bladder, two veins in the neck were bled for leprosy.

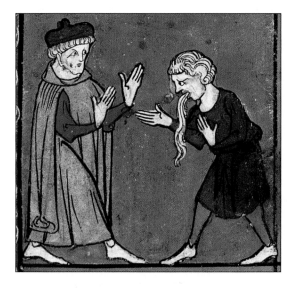

A patient vomiting to get rid of an excess of humours.

Source E

QUESTIONS

1 Draw a chart across two pages as shown below. One page will be headed 'Greek doctors', the second page 'Medieval doctors'. Down the left-hand side write: Examination, Treatments, Code of Conduct, Beliefs about cause of disease. Complete the chart by summarising the main points for each of these categories for Greek doctors and Medieval doctors. Then answer the following question:

Had Medieval doctors made progress since Greek times?

	Greek Doctors	Medieval Doctors
Examination		
Treatments		
Code of conduct		
Beliefs about cause of disease		

Surgery

Surgeons were often regarded as no better than butchers. There were three types: surgeons, barbers and military surgeons.

- Barbers were licensed to cut hair and do minor surgery like pulling teeth, lancing boils, leeching and cupping.

- Surgeons were meant to do blood-letting and more major surgical work although this usually only went as far as manipulating dislocated limbs, setting broken bones, and treating scalds and burns with cauteries.

- Military surgeons had to take more risks with their battered victims of war. Most of the advances made in surgery were made by these surgeons who had to develop new methods on the spot. They were successful, for example, in extracting arrows and cross-bow bolts well.

Surgeons were regarded as inferior to doctors because they did not study at university, but they had to serve an apprenticeship for about six years. They then needed a license from the town guild of surgeons or barbers. There was little difference between surgeons and barbers although a few well-educated and well-paid surgeons did employ barbers as assistants and regarded them as inferior.

The work they could do was limited because of the lack of effective anaesthetics. Alcohol or opium were sometimes used to deaden the pain, but they were not very effective. Because of this, and the danger of loss of blood, they had to work quickly.

The treatment used most, apart from blood-letting, was the cautery. Metal instruments were heated and used to burn away diseased tissue, seal wounds to stop them bleeding, and to remove the cold and moist humours.

Source A

A 13th-century illustration showing different treatments for wounds.

When the cautery is heated then bring it down upon the marked place with one downward stroke with gentle pressure, revolving the cautery. If you see that some bone is exposed, then take away the cautery; otherwise repeat with the same iron till the bone is exposed. Then take a little salt in water, soak some cotton in it, apply to the place, then leave for three days.

Source B

From an 11th-century description of cauterisation.

QUESTIONS

1 What types of surgery were medieval surgeons able to do?

Women and medieval medicine

The Church was very suspicious of women. It saw them as weak, unclean and corrupt creatures. Even Galen had said that women had more of the cold and wet humours and so were less perfect than men, weak-willed and fickle, and more prone to madness! Menstruation showed women to be imperfect because this was the body's way of getting rid of harmful humours. When women stopped menstruating later in life they were seen as full of evil humours. This is one of the reasons why elderly women were often accused of being witches.

The Church and the medical authorities claimed that women were clearly not fit to be doctors. However, before the 14th century they were allowed to train as surgeons and were given licenses, but by the 14th century this had stopped.

Although women could not practise as doctors, they were expected to look after the health of their families. Thousands of ordinary women must have spent a considerable amount of time looking after the old and the sick. They grew herbs for medicine and devised soothing lotions. Treatments were handed on from mother to daughter.

The Church was happy for women to care for their families but it disapproved of the many wise-women and faith healers who sold medicines and other treatments. They used herbs and charms and probably did less harm than many doctors and their excessive bleeding of patients. Most people could not afford to see a qualified doctor and these women probably had more patients than the doctors! Their treatments were often painless and many women preferred to be treated by other women. Women were also employed to care for the sick in hospitals and acted as midwives. So you can see, their role in medicine was not unimportant.

Madame, I have this night taken your medicine, for which I heartily thank you, for it hath done me much good and hath caused the stone to break. But your medicine hath made me piss my bed this night, for which my wife hath sore beaten me.

Source D

Lord Edmund Howard writing to Lady Lisle in 1535 after taking a powder she prepared for him for a bladder stone. The treatment was not totally successful!

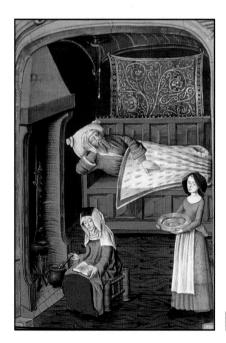

Source E

A woman in the 15th century caring for a sick relative. She is preparing a herbal medicine and consulting a commonplace book where many of the recipes were collected.

Why were monasteries important?

We are back to the Church! There is no getting away from it in the Middle Ages. There were three reasons why monasteries were important to medicine in the Middle Ages:

- they preserved the writings of Hippocrates and Galen
- they built hospitals
- they developed public health systems.

We have already looked at the hospitals they built (see page 63–5).

Preserving Greek and Roman writings

During the Dark Ages after the fall of the Roman Empire monasteries preserved, copied and studied the medical writings of the Greeks and the Romans. Until universities like Salerno began to be built after 1100 the monasteries were the only centres of learning. They kept some Greek and Roman medical ideas alive, and more importantly they kept the books so that centuries later they could be studied again.

Monasteries became medical centres

Many monasteries encouraged the care of the sick. The rule of the Benedictine monks stated that 'the care of the sick is to be placed above and before every other duty'. Monasteries became key medical centres. Most had an infirmary for sick monks and, as we have seen, a separate hospital for the public. At least one of the monks would specialise in caring for the sick monks. He would keep a herb garden and many developed an expert knowledge of all the different types of herbs.

Monasteries and public health

To study the state of public health in the Middle Ages we are going to compare conditions in a monastery with those in a typical town.

Many monasteries were wealthy and had the money to make sure they stayed healthy. They could build water pipes, drains and wash houses. Sources B and C are plans of two monasteries, one was built by the side of a river, the other had its water piped to it.

You can see the reredorter (privies) are built over the river. The laver was a stone trough where the monks washed.

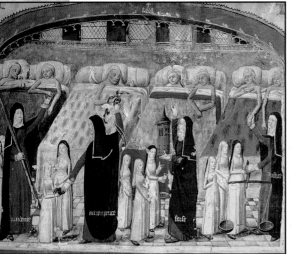

Source A

A medieval illustration showing monks and nuns caring for the sick (two in a bed!).

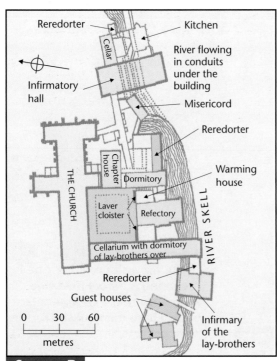

Reredorter — Kitchen
Cellar
River flowing in conduits under the building
Infirmatory hall
Misericord
Reredorter
Chapter house
THE CHURCH
Dormitory
Warming house
Laver cloister — Refectory
RIVER SKELL
Cellarium with dormitory of lay-brothers over
Reredorter
Guest houses
0   30   60
metres
Infirmary of the lay-brothers

Plan of Fountains Abbey.

Source B

Part of the water that fed the fish pond was used to flush the latrines in the necessarium (the privies) and was eventually carried into the town ditch.

The natural wells in the centre cloister and near the fonts – they were used when the main system failed.

The reservoirs – the octafoil basin in the centre with its pair of stand pipes, the smaller one in the cloisters to the right – where part of the water coming from the pipes was stored.

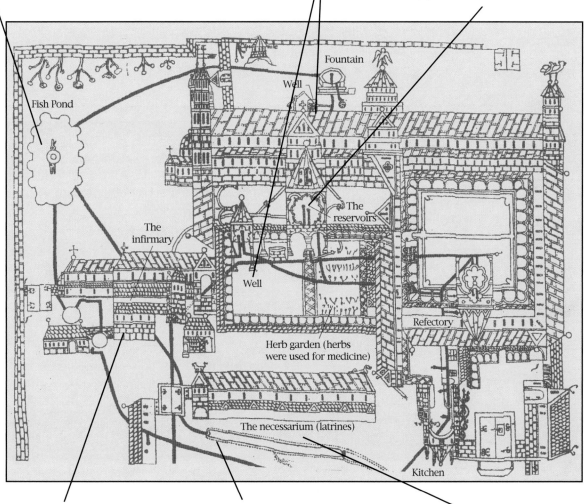

The infirmary buildings – all the monks had to visit here for regular blood-letting, after which they convalesced for a few days.

The drainage system is represented by simple double lines, the rain water was conducted to this system; gutters can be seen around the cloisters on the right and protruding from the main church building.

The necessarium was a large latrine block. It was attached to the monks' communal dormitory.

The water source is about three-quarters of a mile from the bottom of the plan. This water is conveyed through a conduit-house, and by lead pipes, through five settling tanks, through the city wall into the cathedral.

The black lines represent the course of the feeding-pipes.

The water was used to supply the kitchen, the wash rooms, brew houses, bakery and the fish pond.

Source C

Plan of Canterbury Cathedral and its systems of water supply and drainage. It was drawn shortly after the building of the systems in 1153. Parts of the sanitation system are still in use today.

QUESTIONS

1 Explain what features in these monasteries would help keep the monks healthy.

LONDON TODAY

5 May 1340

WHAT A MESS!

Survey reveals rubbish everywhere!

A recent survey of London shows we are all living in what amounts to one big cesspit. The main points of the report include:

- our narrow streets are often blocked by huge dung-heaps
- people living in upper stories have latrines projected over the lane outside – the filth falls onto anyone passing
- only the rich have their own latrines. For the rest of us there are 16 public latrines for the rest of London
- our rubbish should be washed away by rivers like the Wallbrook and the Fleet. However, these are becoming blocked by filth and rubbish because people are building latrines over them. Other people are running pipes from their houses into the rivers
- overflow pipes from cesspools run into the streets.

THE CITY CORPORATION REPLIES

Harry Gysborow, an official from the City Corporation, claimed that they are doing all they can. He said 'We recently prosecuted a man for going to the toilet in the middle of the street. We have passed laws banning people from throwing the contents of bedroom urinals out of their windows. Serjeants of the Channels go round fining people for dumping rubbish in the streets. We also have a team of rakers to take rubbish away in carts and dump it outside the city. The King recently ordered that animals had to be slaughtered outside the city. But we cannot do everything. Traders like butchers and shoe makers dump their rubbish anywhere.'

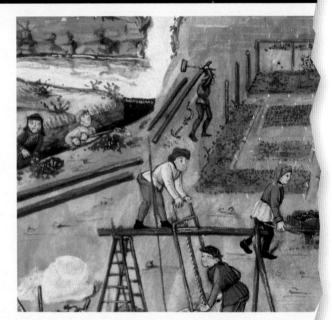

The brave men trying to keep our streams clear of filth.

Problem column

We have had the following letter from Archibald who lives near London Bridge. What should he do?

> Dear Sir
>
> I wish to complain about my neighbour. I live in a cellar with my family. It is damp enough anyway but has been made much worse by our neighbour running a pipe from his house under our cellar. Here the pipe ends and deposits all our neighbour's waste and filth. It is beginning to seep up through our floor. The smell is terrible. What do we do?

George Mud, our intrepid reporter, risks his health and visits the banks of the RiverThames.

It's hell here. It looks like all the butchers of London dump all their offal and entrails along the Thames. I am standing here at low tide. The bank of the river is covered with the entrails of beasts. And to think that many of us get our drinking water from this river!

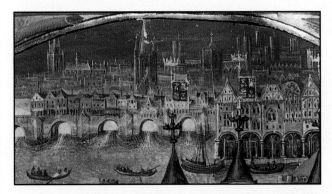

London Bridge – is London over-crowded?

An unfortunate end

Reports are coming through of a death in a cesspool. The unfortunate Richard had just comfortably settled down in his privy when the rotten planks of the floor gave way sending him plunging down into the cesspool. It is reported that the cesspool is so deep there is no chance of Richard being recovered. There have been previous reports that cesspools are becoming favourite places for murderers to dump their victims because the bodies will never be found.

QUESTIONS

1 Keep a diary over three days. Imagine you are living in London. Describe the conditions you live in and the dangers that you face to your health.

EXAM PRACTICE QUESTIONS

(a) Describe the state of public health in medieval towns.

(b) How were Roman towns healthier than medieval towns?

(c) Why were conditions in medieval towns worse than in Roman towns?

CASE STUDY

The Black Death

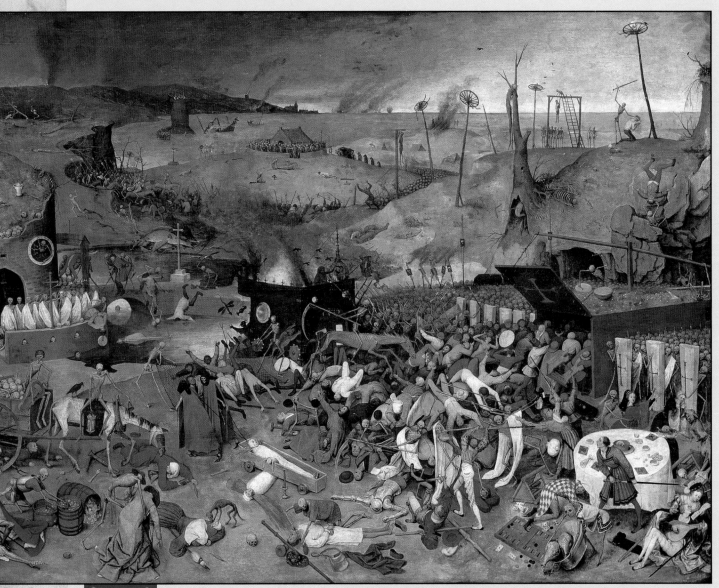

Source A

Look at this picture. It is called 'The Triumph of Death' and shows us how people in the 14th century saw the Black Death (or plague).

Q1 Use Source A to explain what the artist is saying about the Black Death.

The plague had visited Europe off and on since ancient times, but in the 14th century it was devastating. In 1347 it swept through India, Russia, and into Italy. Within a year a quarter of the population of Europe had it. By 1350 nearly half of the population of England was dead. Just think what this meant in human terms – fathers and mothers lost their children, and many children were left without parents.

Nearly every family was affected in some way. This is why people were terrified of the plague and painted pictures like the one in Source A.

How well did people at the time explain and deal with the Black Death? The answers to these questions will tell us a lot about medieval medicine. Later in this book you will be looking at another attack of the plague in the 17th century to see how much progress had been made in understanding it.

Read Source B written in 1353. What does it tell you about (i) the symptoms of the plague, and (ii) its causes?

In the year 1348, in Florence, there occurred a most terrible plague; either because of the influence of the planets or sent from God as a just punishment for our sins. In spite of all means that human foresight could suggest, such as keeping the city clear from filth, and excluding all suspected people, it wreaked incredible havoc.

Swellings appeared on the groin or under the armpits some as big as a small apple, others like an egg. These swellings then spread all over the body. Later on, the symptoms of the disease changed and many people found purple blotches on most parts of the body. These were sure signs, just as the swellings had been, that the victims would die. Few escaped. They usually died the third day after the appearance of the symptoms, the majority without any fever or other complications. The disease grew by being communicated from the sick to the well. Nor was it necessary to talk or even come near the sick. Even touching their clothes or anything they had touched was enough.

Neither the knowledge of medicine nor the power of drugs had any effect. This was either because the disease was fatal or because the doctors, whose number was increased by quacks and woman pretenders, could discover neither the cause nor cure.

Source B

An account of the plague written by Boccaccio in 1353.

Q2 What are the similarities and differences between these two accounts of the Black Death?

Q3 How much did Boccaccio get right?

Q4 How does what you have learned about public health conditions in medieval London help you to understand how the plague spread so easily?

In the filthy conditions of the Middle Ages rats lived side by side with humans. The bacterium that causes the plague infects rats and their fleas. The fleas transmit the infection to other rats when they feed on them. The rats quickly die. The fleas abandon them and move to humans to feed on their blood.

Once bitten, humans have little protection. Cells near the bite die, creating black blisters. Four to six days after the bite buboes, the size of apples, appear. The most usual site of the swellings is in the groin. The victim now has high fever, terrible headache and is delirius. Within ten days of the bite, 60 per cent of those infected will have died. Sometimes those infected developed pneumonic plague and could transmit the disease by coughing on to anyone close by. Pneumonic plague can also be caught from flea faeces from bedding or clothing. The victim coughs blood and dies within two days.

Source C

An account of the plague from a 20th-century book.

CASE STUDY

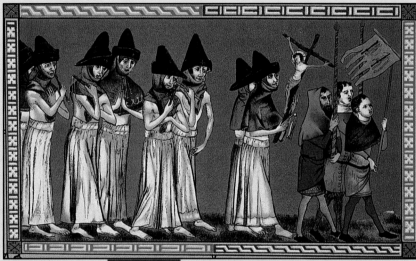

Source D

Flagellants whipping themselves. They believed the plague was a punishment from God for their sins. They are punishing themselves in the hope that God will be more merciful.

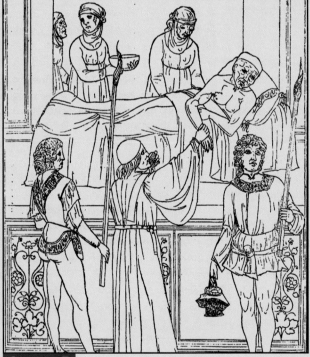

Source E

This woodcut shows a plague patient being treated by a doctor. Can you see the following: the censer used to perfume the air, the burning tapers, a sponge soaked in vinegar. All of these were meant to get rid of bad smells which were spreading the disease.

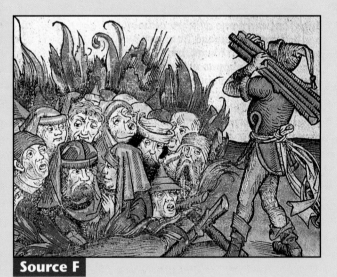

Source F

Jews being burned alive. People often thought that they were deliberately spreading the plague.

To the Lord Mayor of London
An order to cause the human excreta and other filth lying in the streets in the city to be removed with all speed. This is so that no greater cause of death may arise from such smells.

Source G

A letter from King Edward III, 1349.

We command you to let it be known that holy processions are to be held in our cathedral and in every parish church, and that a special prayer be said every day for stopping the plague and pestilence.

Source H

An order issued by the Archbishop of York, 1348.

The distant cause
The first cause of the plague is the position of the heavens. In 1345, at one hour after noon on 20 March, there was a major conjunction of three planets in Aquarius. This caused a deadly corruption of the air.

The near cause
The present plague has happened because evil smells have been mixed with the air and spread by frequent winds. This corrupted air when breathed in penetrates to the heart and destroys the life force.

Hippocrates agreed that if the four seasons do not follow each other in the proper way, then plague will follow. The whole year has been warm and wet and the air is corrupt.

Source I

The King of France asked the doctors at Paris University to report on the causes of the plague in 1348. These are extracts from their report.

Many people have been killed for the cause of the plague is not only the corruption of the air, but the corrupt humours within those who die. You should avoid over-indulgence of food; also avoid baths. These open the pores through which poisonous air can enter. Above all avoid sexual intercourse. In cold or rainy weather you should light fires in your chamber. On going to bed, burn juniper branches so that the smoke and scent fills the room.

If the infected blood is in the armpits, blood should be let from the cardiac vein.

Source J

Written by John of Burgundy in 1365.

Q5 Make a list of the all different causes of the plague you can find in Sources D to J. Do these sources agree with Boccaccio (Source B) about the causes?

Q6 You work for the king in 14th-century London. You have to design a poster that will be pinned up around the city, advising people on how to avoid catching the plague.

Did Islam help or hinder medical development?

While Christian Europe was struggling through the Dark Ages after the fall of the Roman Empire, the new religion of Islam emerged in Arabia in the seventh century. Within a hundred years it had spread through Egypt, Persia, Iraq and even into Spain.

Historians disagree about whether the Muslim religion helped or hindered new developments in medicine. You must decide which of the two following statements you agree with the most.

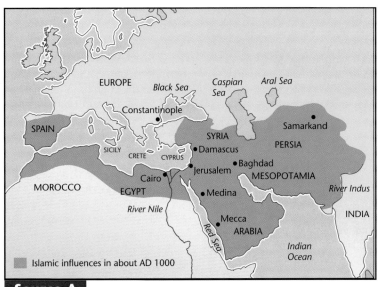

Map of the Arab empire around 1000.

Statement 1

Islam stopped new ideas and methods from being discovered and encouraged doctors to copy Greek ideas.

Statement 2

Islam preserved Greek ideas when they might have been lost. Islamic doctors also added to Greek ideas and were more advanced than doctors in Europe.

Preserving Greek ideas

Muslims had a great respect for learning, and translated, preserved, studied and added to Greek and Roman writings. In Baghdad, in the eighth century, Greek medical writings, especially Galen's, were collected and translated into Arabic. Muslim writers added their own commentaries. If it were not for these writers, many Greek ideas might have been lost for ever. Around 1,100 of these books were translated into Latin and reintroduced Greek ideas back into Europe. Many of these books were still being used in Europe 800 years later!

Three important Islamic writers

Rhazes (850–923)

Rhazes wrote 237 books on medicine. Much of his work was copied from, or based on, the theories of Hippocrates and Galen and he was responsible for bringing much Greek medicine to the Arabic world. He wrote 'he who studies the works of the Ancients, gains the experience of their work as if he himself had lived thousands of years spent on investigation'. He followed the Theory of the Four Humours and used blood-letting a lot.

However, he did criticise doctors who followed Galen uncritically – 'all that is written in books is worth much less than the experience of a wise doctor'. He used his own observations and recorded his own cases. He is important because he produced the first descriptions of smallpox and measles. You can see from Source B how exact his descriptions are.

The eruption of smallpox is preceded by continued fever, pains in the back, itching in the nose and delirium in sleep. Then acute prickling is felt and this goes all over the body, the cheeks go red and the eyes are inflamed. The patient has a sense of heaviness, he sneezes, yawns, feels pain in the throat and chest, and breathes and coughs with difficulty. Note that feeling restless, sick and troubled is more frequent in chicken-pox, while pains in the back are features of the smallpox. The physical signs of measles are nearly the same as those of smallpox but the pains in the back are less. The rash of measles usually appears at once, but the rash of smallpox returns. When the pustules appear, care must be taken of the eyes. Very small white pustules coming into contact with each other are dangerous.

Source B

Rhazes.

Ibn Sina (980–1037) (or Avicenna, as he was known in Europe)

Ibn Sina produced 100 books. These were copies of, and commentaries on, Greek writings. His medical encylopaedia was used in Europe to train doctors until the 17th century, and he was mainly responsible for bringing Greek writings to Europe.

The greatest care must be taken during surgery to prevent infection, because surgery is impossible if the wound is infected.

Source C

Ibn Sina.

Ibn al-Nafis (1200–1288)

Ibn al-Nafis corrected Galen about the heart. His discovery (see Source D) was made 300 years before the same discovery was made in Europe.

Ibn al-Nafis.

When the blood in the right cavity of the heart has become thin, it must be transferred into the left cavity. But there is no passage between these cavities. It neither contains a visible passage, nor does it contain an invisible passage as Galen thought. It must be that the blood is passed to the lung, to mix with air. The blood then passes to the left side of the heart.

Source D

Ideas about disease

Muslims believed that illness was given by Allah as punishment for a person's sins. They believed that prayer might lead to cures, but they also believed in the Four Humours and thought that Allah cured people through doctors. This meant that people were encouraged to use doctors. Dissection of the human body was banned because of their belief in an afterlife. This meant that they added little to the Greek writings on anatomy and they relied on Galen for much of their knowledge.

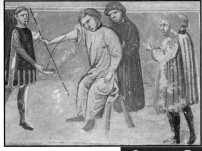

Source E

Blood-letting from one of Ibn Sina's books.

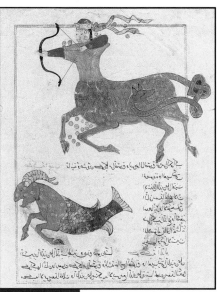

Source F

Drawings of the star constellations Sagittarius and Capricorn from a 14th-century book about how to use stars in diagnosis and treatment.

Methods and treatment

Diagnosis

Doctors reached a diagnosis by examining the patient's behaviour, products of the body such as excreta and urine, swellings, the intensity and the location of pain, the patient's pulse, and the position of the stars.

Examination of urine was very important. Its colour, smell and taste was also used to decide on the right treatment.

Surgery

Surgery was looked down on and was carried out by untrained people. Their limited knowledge of the body also held them back. Cauterisation was the commonest form of surgery and they gave detailed instructions on how to use it to open abscesses, burn skin tumours, cleanse wounds and staunch blood flow. Anaesthetics were also developed – patients held a sponge soaked in drugs against their nose. The design of scissors, syringes and forceps was also improved.

Drugs, antiseptics and anaesthetics

Islamic doctors had a lot of knowledge of new plants and substances from animals that could be used in medicine, like musk and myrrh and bezoar. Laudanum was used as a pain killer and alcohol as an antiseptic. Islamic doctors also set up the first pharmacies.

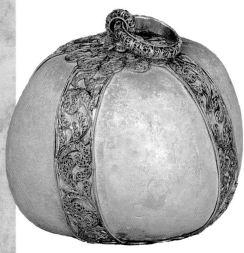

Source G

A Bezoar stone. This was found in the stomachs of goats and was thought to have miraculous powers against poisons.

No slaughtering should take place in the market, except in the closed slaughterhouses, and the blood and the refuse should be taken outside the market.

Cheese should only be sold in small leather bottles which should be washed and cleaned every day.

Source H

Market laws from 12th-century Seville (a Spanish city under Islamic control).

Public health and hospitals

The large Islamic cities like Cairo and Baghdad were no cleaner or filthier than those in Europe. They suffered from the same diseases, for example in 1347–9 Cairo, the world's second largest city with 500,000 people, lost half of its population to the plague. However, Islam taught that people should keep themselves clean e.g. bath once a week and regularly brush their teeth.

Islam also taught that the sick should be looked after and hospitals should be built for them. Hospitals were one of the great achievements of Islam. They were not run by the Church and concentrated on medical treatment for the sick rather than on prayer. They were more advanced than those in Europe, and were open to all – rich and poor – and provided a retirement home for the old and infirm. The hospital in Cairo had separate wards for different diseases, a separate ward for convalescents, a surgery, a pharmacy, library and lecture rooms. When patients went home they were given money so didn't have to return to work immediately.

QUESTIONS

1 For each of the following categories briefly write down examples of how Islamic medicine and Western medicine were similar or different: using Greek ideas, ideas about disease, knowledge of the body, how doctors worked, treatments, surgery, public health.

2 Read the two statements at the beginning of this section. Explain which statement you agree with the most.

HELP YOUR REVISION

Factors

- The fall of the Roman Empire and weak governments.
- Christianity – a good or bad influence on medicine?
- Islam – a good or bad influence on medicine?
- Galen – a good or bad influence on medicine?

Ideas about disease

- Spirits and magic.
- A punishment by God.
- The position of the planets.
- The Four Humours.
- Bad air and smells.

Other important points

- Regression after the Romans.
- The building of Medieval hospitals.
- Women played an important role.
- Doctors being trained but surgeons regarded as inferior.
- Poor public health.

EXAM PRACTICE QUESTIONS

Before attempting this question go through the complete section on the Middle Ages and make two lists: one of all the ways the Christian Church helped medicine develop; the second of all the ways it hindered the development of medicine. These lists will give you plenty of examples to use in answering this question.

(a) Describe three ways in which the Christian Church helped the development of medieval medicine.

(b) Explain how the Christian Church hindered the development of medieval medicine.

(c) Did the Christian Church hinder the development of medicine more than it helped? Explain your answer.

What has happened so far?

	Ideas about disease	Treatments
Prehistoric	Spirits cause disease.	Treated simple surface wounds. Spirits used for other illnesses. Trephinning.
Egyptians	Gods cause disease. Disease caused by blockage of channels in body.	Good treatment of external injuries. Drugs used. Doctors examine patients. Simple surgery. Purging e.g. blood-letting used. Individuals kept clean but no public health. Praying to Gods. Wearing amulets.
Greeks	Asclepios and Temple medicine. Theory of the Four Humours.	Attending an Asclepeion. Purging. Clinical method of observation. Healthy lifestyle and diet. Individuals kept clean, no public health. Simple surgery.
Romans	Gods – Asclepios. No new theories – ideas about the Four Humours were accepted. Prefer prevention to cure.	Public health developed. Surgery developed. Galen's use of Opposites.
The Middle Ages	Magic and spirits. Punishment from God. Four Humours. Astrology. Bad air and smells.	Prayer, charms. Development of hospitals. Purging very important. Not much progress in surgery or public health. Islamic development of drugs and hospitals.

Individuals	Factors	Rate of change
	Lifestyle as hunter gatherers, later as farmers.	Very slow over 100,000s of years. Speeded up a little when people became farmers.
	Isolation led to stability but then no new influences so there was stagnation. Writing – kept medical records. Religion – led to mummifying but dissection was banned. Religion also made them keep clean.	Some change at first, then little change.
Hippocrates	Greek philosophy – the Four Elements. Religion – dissection was banned, and there was little knowledge of anatomy and physiology.	Little progress in knowledge of the body, but much in ideas. The Four Humours was a big step forward as it was the first explicit natural explanation.
Galen – develops knowledge of anatomy and physiology.	They copied the Greeks. The needs of the Army. Christianity – banned dissection. Engineering and building skills important.	No development in ideas but important practical advances in public health and surgery.
Galen Ibn Sina Ibn al-Nafis	Fall of Rome. Impact of Christian Church and monasteries was good and bad. Galen's influence. Islamic religion.	Slow development under Anglo-Saxons. Islam preserved the ancient knowledge, but Galen's ideas prevented much progress. Overall regression since Roman times.

What happened in the Medical Renaissance?

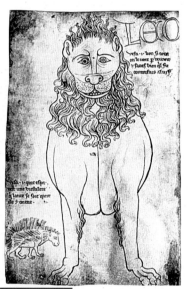

Source A

A drawing of a lion and a porcupine from 1235.

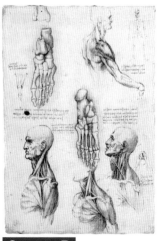

Source B

Many books will tell you that the development of medicine was helped by the Renaissance. But what was the Renaissance, and how did it help medicine?

What was the Renaissance?

New interest in the Greeks

The Renaissance took place in western Europe roughly between 1400 and 1600. The word means rebirth – a rebirth of interest in what the Greeks and Romans had written, drawn and built.

As you have seen, Greek medicine dominated medieval medicine. However, in the Renaissance there was a new love of all things that were Greek. Scholars were worried that Arabic and medieval translations of Greek writings were not accurate. They went back to the original Greek sources. They thought that if they did this they would find the eternal truths about medicine that the Greeks had discovered and which were lost in the Middle Ages. New translations of Hippocrates and Galen were made. Between 1500 and 1600, 590 new editions of Galen were published. At first Galen's ideas were followed to the letter.

However, this new interest in the Greeks led people to take an interest in the world around them. Like the Greeks they began to ask questions about how nature worked. They observed nature carefully. They started to find things out for themselves rather than simply believing everything the Greeks said. And when they began to study the human body in this way, Galen's mistakes became obvious.

Art and anatomy

In the Middle Ages most art was religious – what was important was the story it told not how realistically the people and nature had been drawn. Illustrations of humans were simply copied from earlier drawings with no attempt to study the real thing.

During the Renaissance, artists began to try to draw the body accurately. To do this they realised that knowledge of the different parts of the body was needed. Leonardo da Vinci dissected bodies and produced a series of anatomical notebooks with detailed drawings of parts of the body. Drawings like these began to appear in anatomy textbooks. Compare the drawings in Sources A and B.

Galen had had to use animals. But he always said that you should look at the body for yourself rather than just copying what was in books. This meant if people followed what Galen said they would, sooner or later, see his mistakes.

Drawings by Leonardo da Vinci from around 1510.

Science and technology

There were also important developments in science and technology. One of these was the invention of the printing press. In the Middle Ages every book had been written by hand. When Greek books were copied in this way mistakes were often made. In 1450 Johann Gutenberg invented the first printing press. This meant that thousands of copies of a book could be easily printed. New ideas could now be spread all over Europe.

Other developments included mechanical pumps, the invention of microscopes and Leonardo da Vinci even made drawings of flying machines and submarines. The introduction of gunpowder into Europe from China led to cannons and guns being developed.

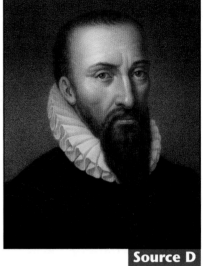

Source D

Paré developed new ideas in surgery.

QUESTIONS

1 Can you work out ways in which the Renaissance would help developments in medicine?

How did all this help medicine?

The development of medicine at this time was led by three men – Andreas Vesalius, Ambroise Paré and William Harvey. As you read about their work you must decide how important each was. Were they great men or did they make their discoveries simply because they were living at the time when new ideas were common?

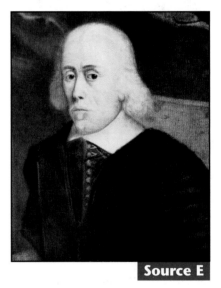

Source E

Harvey discovered that blood circulates around the body.

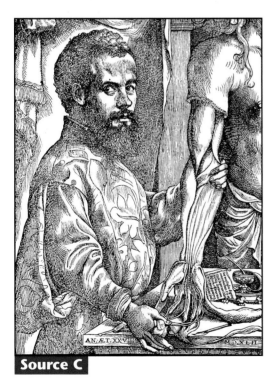

Source C

Vesalius made important discoveries about the structure of the human body.

Andreas Vesalius (1514-64)

Biography

Born in Brussels, Vesalius studied medicine at the University of Paris. He moved to Padua University where he taught surgery and anatomy. Here dissections were encouraged and artists were already making careful drawings of the body. As he carried out more dissections and produced anatomical drawings for his students, Vesalius began to realise that Galen had made mistakes. He taught his students that anatomy could only be learned by direct observation of the body rather than by reading Galen.

In 1539 Vesalius acquired a large supply of bodies of executed criminals and began the work that led to his great book. In 1543 (when he was only 28) he published *The Fabric of the Human Body*. This, through its writing and drawings, gave a complete guide to the human body. It also showed where Galen had been wrong.

There was much opposition to his ideas from those who believed that Galen could not be wrong. When Vesalius supported his ideas by showing his drawings the opposition claimed that humans must have changed over the twelve hundred years since Galen! Upset by this Vesalius left Padua and spent the rest of his life working as a doctor for the Emperor Charles V.

Why was *The Fabric of the Human Body* so important?

It was important because it showed Galen was wrong and corrected some of his mistakes

Vesalius's book was the first proper account of human anatomy because it was based on human dissection – no animals were used. It showed that Galen had made mistakes in the following areas:

- The human breast-bone has three segments not seven
- The human jawbone is not made of two bones
- The human liver does not have lobes
- The septum in the heart does not have invisible pores in it. Galen had claimed that blood flowed from the right to the left ventricle of the heart through these pores.

Vesalius's book did the unthinkable. It showed that Galen was wrong. Once this had been done others were willing to test Galen's ideas for themselves.

It was important because of the methods it told doctors to use

Dissections were carried out in the Middle Ages to illustrate what Galen had written but Vesalius used dissection to test what Galen had written. In his book he stresses that to learn about the body doctors must carry out human dissections. The only way they can learn is by observing for themselves. His book is important because it shows doctors and anatomists the way forward. It gives them the method by which they would make many further discoveries about the human body in the future.

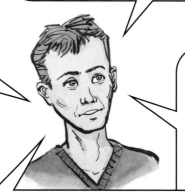

It was important because of the printing press

Thousands of copies of Vesalius's book could be printed and sent all over Europe, quickly spreading his new ideas. The printing press also meant that as no copying had to be done no mistakes were made. Vesalius's writings and the illustrations were printed exactly. In the past drawings had often been copied incorrectly.

It was important because of the use it makes of drawings

It contained realistic and technically correct drawings, which showed dissected parts of the body. These drawings were closely integrated with the writing. One helped explain the other. Especially important was the series of drawings of 'muscle-men' at different stages of dissection. These drawings were so important to Vesalius that he drew some of them himself and supervised the printing of the engravings. For the first time doctors had accurate drawings of the human body.

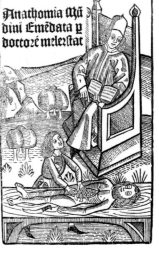

Source A

An illustration of a dissection before Vesalius in 1316. The teacher sits in a chair and reads from Galen while his assistant dissects the body.

Vesalius conducts a public anatomy. The fact that this drawing appeared at the front of Vesalius's book shows the importance he attached to doctors carrying out dissections for themselves and learning from what they saw.

The three robed figures represent Galen and other Greek figures. They are now on a level with Vesalius. He is no longer looking up to them. The dog and the monkey represent the animals that Galen used for anatomy.

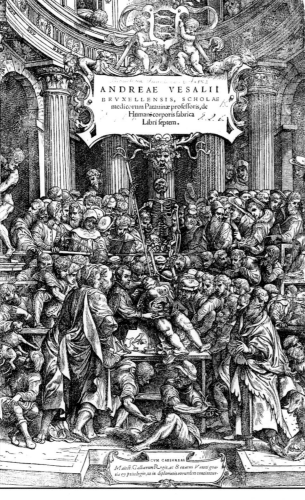

Vesalius is not sitting in a chair using demonstrators, he is actually doing the dissection himself. The unemployed demonstrators are shown quarrelling under the table.

The bones of the skeleton would be constantly referred to during the dissection.

The spectators stood on wooden stands.

Vesalius is surrounded by his students.

Source B

This illustration was placed right at the beginning of *The Fabric of the Human Body.*

QUESTIONS

1   You have read about four reasons why Vesalius's book was important. Write one sentence about each, summing up its main points.

Which reason do you think was the most important?

2   Study Sources A and B. Explain why Vesalius had the illustration in Source B placed at the beginning of his book.

Biography

Paré was born in a small village in France. He was apprenticed to a barber-surgeon when he was 13 and then worked as an assistant-surgeon at the Hôtel-Dieu, the chief hospital in Paris. In 1536 Paré started working as a surgeon for the French army.

It was while working with the army that he made his greatest discoveries. In 1562 Paré was appointed by King Charles IX as his chief surgeon and in 1564 published his most important book, *Ten Books of Surgery*.

Paré was not educated at university and was always looked down on by surgeons working at universities. In 1585 he published his *Apologie and Treatise* to defend his ideas. By the time of his death he was the most famous surgeon in Europe.

Ambroise Paré (1510–90) and advances in surgery

Surgery before Paré

When Paré started working with the army the treatments used were basic and very painful.

Amputations

Gunpowder was first used in Europe in the 14th century. This led to the development of guns and cannons. Many soldiers were so badly injured they had their limbs amputated. This left spurting arteries hanging out. The area around the amputation was cauterised – a red-hot iron was used to burn the flesh. The skin was then pulled over the oozing stump and was stitched with large heavy needles. This was all done to prevent infection and stop the bleeding. It was agonizing – some soldiers died from shock while it was being done.

Gunshot wounds

The method used to treat gunshot wounds was just as barbaric. The new guns fired stone or metal shot, and later bullets, which inflicted the most horrible wounds. The shot or bullet was cut out with a razor. Meanwhile, boiling oil was kept bubbling in metal pots. A cloth was dropped into the oil. The cloth dripping with boiling oil was thrust deep into the wound, which was then bandaged. This was meant to burn away the poison which they thought was produced by the gunpowder. And remember, they had no effective anaesthetics in those days!

So patients suffered – from pain and fever, they were disfigured or crippled, and many died.

The importance of Paré

Paré is important for four reasons.

1. Ligatures instead of red hot irons

As early as 1552 Paré began using ligatures instead of cauterising. In his *Ten Books of Surgery,* Paré recommended replacing cauterising with tying the veins and arteries with ligatures (silk threads) after an amputation to stop the bleeding.

This was not a new idea. Other writers had suggested it but Paré worked out the practical details. However, ligatures were not widely used for a long time. There were three reasons for this: 53 ligatures were necessary for a thigh amputation; a method was needed to control the flow of blood until the blood vessels could all be tied; and the threads often spread infection in the wound.

2. Soothing ointments instead of burning oils.

In this conflict there were many wounded on both sides with all sorts of weapons but chiefly with bullets. I will tell the truth, I was not very expert at that time in surgery, neither was I used to dressing wounds made by gunshot. I had read in Jean de Vigo that wounds made by gunshot were poisoned so for their cure it was necessary to cauterise them with scalding hot oil. I knew that this would cause great pain and I was determined to see whether the other surgeons used any other methods of dressing these wounds. I observed that all of them used this method. This encouraged me to do the same.

By chance, and because of the great numbers that were injured, I ran out of oil. I was forced to use a mixture of egg yolks, oil of roses and turpentine. I could not sleep all that night because I feared that the next day I should find them dead because I had not killed the poison with boiling oil. I rose early in the morning and visited my patients. To my surprise I found that those treated with the ointment had slept and only had a little pain. Their wounds were not inflamed. The others that were burnt with the oil were feverish, in much pain, and their wounds were swollen. I decided never to cauterise gunshot wounds again.

Source A

Paré writing about his time with the French army in 1536. He wrote this account in 1545.

4. Artificial Limbs

In several of his books Paré included drawings of artifical limbs. He had many of these made and used them for the numerous injured soldiers he treated who had lost limbs.

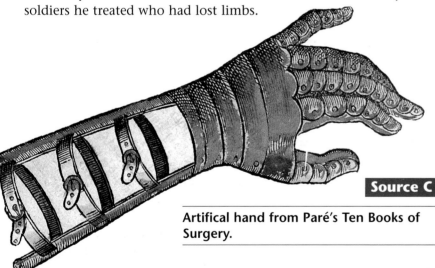

Source C

Artifical hand from Paré's Ten Books of Surgery.

3. Experiments used to test ideas

In 1566 a visitor to King Charles IX brought a gift – a bezoar stone. These stones, from the stomachs of goat-like animals, were supposed to have magical properties and to cure all poisons (see page 86). The King asked Paré whether it was possible for one drug to kill all poisons. Paré replied it was not because different poisons work in different ways. When the visitor insisted that bezoar did work Paré suggested they test it in an experiment. In Source B we have Paré's account of this experiment.

A cook was brought by the jailor who was to have been hanged for stealing two silver dishes. The King desired to know whether he would take the poison on condition that if the bezoar should free him from death then he should have his life. The cook answered cheerfully that he was willing to take a chance and had poison given him and then after the poison some of the bezoar. A while after he began to vomit, and to cry out that his inwards parts were burnt with fire.

An hour after, I found him on the ground like a beast upon hands and feet, with his tongue thrust out of his mouth, his eyes fiery, vomiting, and blood flowing forth from his ears, nose and mouth.

At length he died with great pain, seven hours after taking the poison. The King commanded – burn the bezoar.

Source B

QUESTIONS

1 Paré had his critics. This was because he had not studied medicine at university. He was only a surgeon, and he had learnt surgery in a practical way. One person who would have defended Paré was Vesalius. They lived in Paris at the same time. Imagine you are Vesalius. Write a defence of Paré and his methods. Source D, written by Paré replying to one of his critics, might help you.

How dare you teach me surgery, you who have done nothing all your life but look at books. Surgery is learned with the hand and the eye. All you know is how to talk your head off, sitting comfortably in a chair.

Source D

William Harvey (1578–1657) and the circulation of blood

Biography William Harvey was born in 1578 in Folkestone, England and studied medicine at Padua. Here he was taught by Fabricius, who encouraged his students to dissect animals to discover how organs worked. Fabricius also wrote about the valves in the veins allowing the blood to flow in only one direction. This was to be important in Harvey's theory about the circulation of blood.

Harvey worked in London as a doctor. He later became a physician to kings James I and Charles I. By 1625 he had become convinced that blood circulates around the body.

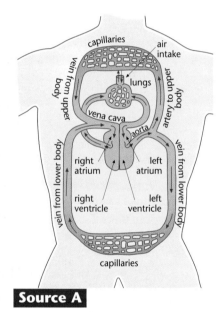

Source A

Study Source A. It shows what we know today about how blood moves around our bodies.

1 **The left ventricle of the heart contracts – blood is forced out into the great artery.**
2 **The blood passes into smaller arteries and then into the capillaries.**
3 **It returns to the heart through the veins and the vena cava.**
4 **The blood then enters the right ventricle of the heart and moves on to the lungs.**
5 **In the lungs it is oxygenated before returning to the left ventricle.**

Harvey was the first person to work this out. How did he do it?

Step 1 The story so far

Doctors had always known that blood was important but it took a long time to figure out exactly how blood worked. However, Harvey did not have to start at the beginning. As you can see, doctors just before Harvey were beginning to develop new ideas about blood.

Give each of the following marks out of 10 for how much they might have helped Harvey.

- Galen wrongly claimed that blood passed from one side of the heart to the other through pores in the septum. He also believed that the body used up blood and that the liver constantly made new blood.

- Ibn al-Nafis (1210–88) said blood did not go through the septum but through the lungs. However, few people in Europe had heard of him.

- Andreas Vesalius (1514–64) claimed that blood did not go through the septum. He could not go further than this. His books were well known but not everyone accepted his ideas.

- Realdo Columbo (1516–59) followed Vesalius as Professor at Padua. We know Harvey copied the passage in Source B from one of Columbo's books.

- Fabricius (1533–1619) taught Harvey. He showed him that there were valves in the veins.

Everyone thinks that there is a way open for the blood to pass from the right ventricle to the left. But they err by a long way, for the blood is carried to the lung through the pulmonary artery and in the lung it is refined, and then together with the air it is brought through the pulmonary vein to the left ventricle of the heart.

Source B

All these different ideas simply created confusion. Some of them were beginning to correct Galen's findings but no one had managed to put the whole story of blood together.

Step 2 Water pumps!

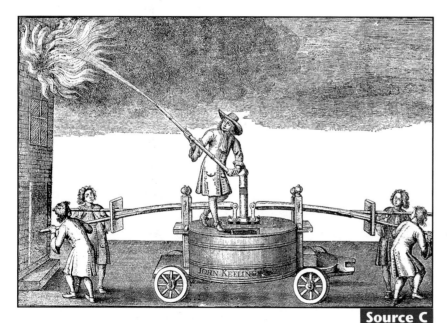

Source C

A water pump being used in the 17th century to fight fire. In 1615 the following description of a fire pump was written: 'There are two valves within it, one below to open when the handle is lifted up and to shut when it is down, and another to open to let out the water.'

By Harvey's time mechanical pumps were in use in London as fire pumps. He would have seen these pumps in action. It is possible that Harvey got the idea of the heart being a pump from these machines. Galen would never have thought of this because he had never seen a pump.

Step 3 Some brilliant thinking and a clever experiment

Once he had decided that the heart pumps blood out into the arteries Harvey was faced with another problem. The amount of blood pumped into the arteries each hour (the heart beats many times in an hour) would be more blood than the body contains. Harvey's answer was a stroke of genius – 'I began to consider if blood had a movement in a circle.'

Harvey had already noticed that there were flaps on the inside of veins and arteries. He realised that these flaps must be valves which made blood flow through the veins in one direction (towards the heart), and in the other direction through the arteries (away from the heart).

Remember:

- Fabricius (who taught Harvey) had already noticed the valves, although he did not know what they were for.
- Harvey had seen valves being used in fire pumps.

To test his idea Harvey carried out the experiment shown in Source D.

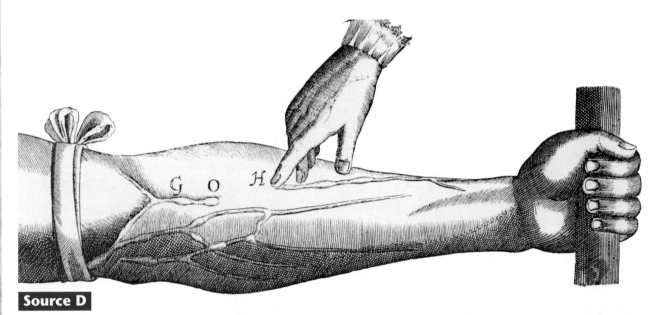

Source D

1 The upper arm was bandaged to restrict the flow of blood.
2 This made the valves visible (G, O, H).
3 Harvey pushed his finger along a vein from one valve to the next in a direction away from the heart e.g. O to H.
4 The vein between O and H emptied of blood.
5 It stayed empty because the valve O did not allow blood to flow back.

Harvey's discovery is one of the most important in the history of medicine. It gave doctors a new map of how the body worked. Without it surgeons today would not be able to carry out blood transfusions or any complicated internal surgery. However, there was one piece of this map that Harvey did not discover. Look again at Source A on page 96. You can see that capillaries carry blood from the ends of the arteries to the beginnings of the veins. Harvey did not see these capillaries because there were no microscopes good enough to make the capillaries visible.

QUESTIONS

1 Copy the grid below. In each column, write a sentence or two explaining how the factors helped Harvey.

Earlier ideas	Harvey's genius	Water pumps	Use of experiments

Now explain which factor was the most important in helping Harvey.

HELP YOUR REVISION

Factors

■ The Renaissance helped developments in medicine. It encouraged careful, first-hand observation of the human body and the challenging of old ideas. But the advances made were also due to three brilliant individuals.

■ Vesalius used Galen's methods of investigation – but showed Galen had made mistakes. He produced the most complete account of the structure of the human body.

■ Paré replaced the cautery iron with ligatures, used soothing ointments instead of burning oil, tested bezoar, and developed artificial limbs.

■ Harvey used experiments to show that blood circulates around the body.

Ideas about disease

■ None of these men came up with new ideas about the cause of disease.

Other important points

■ The development of pumps, the invention of printing, and the warfare of this time, all helped developments in medicine.

■ Paré was helped by chance. (Remember, he ran out of oil.)

■ Although Vesalius, Paré and Harvey all made important advances, did these advances lead to patients receiving better treatments?

EXAM PRACTICE QUESTIONS

(a) Describe the main features of Vesalius's work.

(b) Explain how Paré was helped in his work by chance.

(c) Who is the more important in the history of medicine, Vesalius or Harvey?

Did things change much after the Medical Renaissance?

Vesalius, Paré and Harvey all made important discoveries, but did these lead to immediate changes?

Here you are going to investigate how far ideas about the causes of disease and methods of treatment changed by studying:

- the Great Plague of 1665
- the death of Charles II, King of England, in 1685.

CASE STUDY

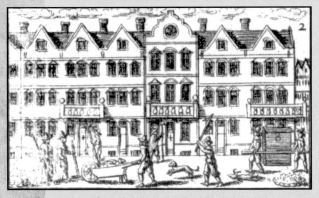

Drawing 1

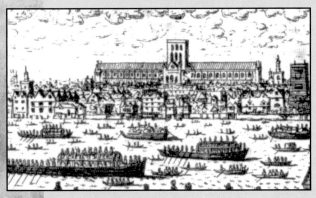

Drawing 2

The Great Plague of 1665

You will remember studying the Black Death of the 1340s. After that date there were smaller outbreaks of the plague in Europe up to the 18th century. The most serious outbreak in England was in 1665. In London 60,000 people were killed (there were only 500,000 people living in London at the time). You are going to study what was done to try to stop the plague from spreading. From this information you can work out how people thought the plague was spread. You are then going to compare this with what was done at the time of the Black Death to see if there had been any progress.

The drawings on this page come from a plague broadsheet published in London in 1666. They show what was happening in London at the time and give lots of clues about what was being done to stop the plague from spreading. Look at the drawings and then match each description to the correct drawing.

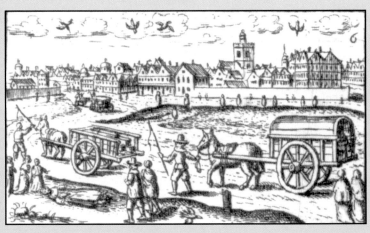

Drawing 4

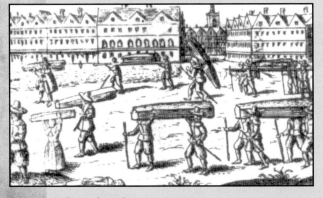

Drawing 3

Description A

You can see the Examiners checking which houses had plague victims in. When they found such a house it was shut up. Nobody in the house was allowed to leave and a red cross was painted on the door. This isolated the sick and those who were in danger, which would stop them infecting other people. The words 'Lord have Mercy upon us' were also drawn on the door. Some people believed dogs were spreading the plague. You can see dogs being killed – dog-killers were appointed to do this. Every householder had to keep the street in front of their house clean. Rakers were employed to take away rubbish. You can also see a fire in the street. Some people believed bad air was responsible for the plague – it was believed the fire would purify the air.

Description B

This family clearly has several people suffering from the plague. It looks as if at least one person has already died. The women with the staffs are probably searchers. Their job was to find people who had died of the plague and to report this. A doctor then examined the body to make sure they had died of the plague. The figure on the right looks like a doctor giving a patient some medicine.

Description C

So many people died that most of them were buried in mass pits like this one. They were dug outside the city and had to be at least six feet deep. People believed that infection from the bodies could make the air go bad – thus spreading the plague. If you look carefully you can see birds dropping down dead from the sky. They have just flown into some bad air and been killed.

Description D

This drawing shows people leaving London any way they can. Here they are fleeing by boats on the River Thames.

Did people understand the plague better in the 17th century than in the 14th century? You are going to write an essay on this. First, it will be helpful to make some notes. You will need to go back to the work you did on the Black Death.

Q1 Make lists of what people thought was spreading the plague in (i) the 14th century (ii) the 17th century. Find reasons that are the same, and those that are different. Now compare what they did to stop the plague spreading. Were they doing the same things in the 17th century as they did in the 14th century?

Q2 You can now use the information you have gathered to answer the following question: Did people in the 17th century understand the plague better than people did in the 14th century? Explain your answer.

CASE STUDY

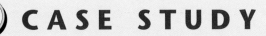

The death of Charles II

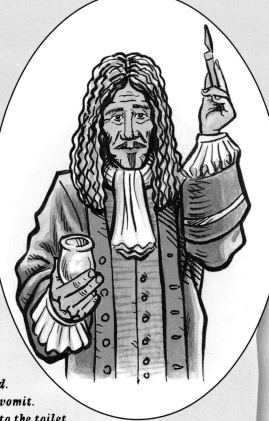

On 2 February 1685 Charles II, 54 years old, suffered a stroke. He lost his speech and had convulsions. At least twelve doctors came to treat him. As you will see they seem to have used every treatment they could think of. None of them did Charles much good. He died four days later.

Read the following description of the treatments. Then copy the chart at the bottom on the opposite page and complete it.

February 2

The first thing the King's Physicians did was to open a vein in his right arm and draw off sixteen ounces of blood. They then made cuts on his shoulders and used cupping-glasses to draw off another eight ounces of blood.

The King was then given a strong emetic to make him vomit. They then squirted liquid up his bottom to make him go to the toilet.

It was clear that none of this was doing him any good so they shaved his head and applied blistering agents.

February 3

Another ten ounces of blood were drawn off. Throughout the day Charles had to take what they called 'Sacred Tincture' (Holy Medicine). To help him with a pain in his throat he was given a soothing gargle made from barley water and syrup.

February 4

The King was getting worse. He was given a laxative and then 40 drops of a medicine described as 'spirit of human skull' (it was probably meant to have magical powers).

February 5

Charles was given some Peruvian Bark.

February 6

The doctors were now getting desperate. Every other hour they gave him small amounts of Oriental Bezoar Stone. He died later in the day.

Treatment	Idea about causes of disease (explain how you know)	Idea – supernatural or natural?	New or old idea? (explain how you know)

Q1 Use the work you have done on the Great Plague and the death of Charles II to explain how very little the Renaissance changed:
(i) ideas about the causes of disease, and
(ii) methods of treatment.

Q2 Why did the work of Vesalius and Harvey bring about so little change?

The centuries of progress

For the exam you will need to know:

☑ Reasons why there was so much progress in this period

It can be argued that the 19th and 20th centuries are the most important centuries in the history of medicine. Just look at the chart opposite. It summarises some of the main advances. We are going to be looking at advances in four areas. See if you can place the advances into the correct area: the fight against germs, surgery, public health and hospitals.

Industrial cities sprang up – overcrowded and filthy. Diseases spread e.g. cholera, creating pressure for public health reforms

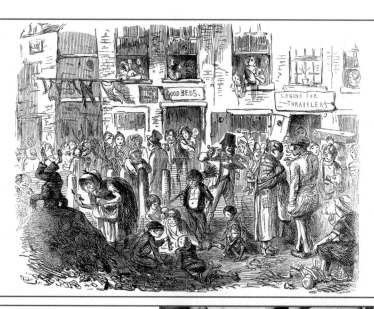

New industries developed new and better materials cheaply – e.g. better glass led to more powerful microscopes. Heart-lung machines were developed helping complicated surgery, and artifical hearts were manufactured.

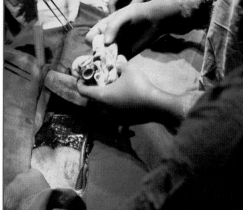

Understanding of chemistry improved, allowing development of new drugs.

Several important wars in this period led to improvements in medicine e.g. plastic surgery, development of penicillin.

In 1867 and 1884 the working classes were given the vote for the first time. This meant that they could put pressure on governments to improve public health. Public health reforms followed.

Individuals such as Florence Nightingale and James Simpson made important contributions.

The end of the 18th century	The end of the 19th century	20th century
Knew germs existed but did not know they caused disease	Knew germs caused disease, and also knew which germs caused which diseases. This led to the development of drugs to fight some diseases. Vaccinations were also developed to protect people against diseases.	Effective drugs such as penicillin developed. Some diseases like smallpox wiped out, but some diseases becoming resistant to drugs. New diseases such as AIDS appearing
Only simple surgery could take place because the problems of pain, infection and bleeding had not been overcome.	Antiseptics and anaesthetics were developed allowing complicated operations to take place.	Advanced surgery taking place e.g. organ transplants, keyhole surgery.
Living conditions, especially in the new towns, were appalling. Public health was almost non-existent, spreading diseases such as cholera and typhoid.	Local councils and governments began to introduce public health reforms which increased life expectancy. But still much poverty and low life expectancy among the poor.	NHS provided health care for all. Nearly all houses have clean piped water and sewage disposal. Rapid rise in life expectancy. But NHS under pressure and under-funded.
There was no proper training for nurses, many of whom were of a low standard. Hospitals were terrible places that the rich stayed clear of.	Schools for training nurses were set up. Proper standards were established. Hospitals were slowly improving.	National network of hospitals established under the NHS providing free care. But hospitals could not cope with rising demand because of more elderly people and because of new expensive treatments. Shortage of doctors and nurses.

The fight against germs

For the exam you will need to know:

☑ How Jenner discovered vaccination

☑ How Pasteur proved germ theory right and other theories wrong

☑ How Pasteur discovered how vaccination works

☑ How Koch developed ways to study germs and proved that each disease is caused by a different kind of germ

☑ How the first drugs like Salverson 606 were developed

☑ How antibiotics like penicillin were developed.

One of the reasons why so much progress was made in the 19th century was the discovery that germs cause disease. We have seen the many ways people tried to explain disease, e.g. the Four Humours, miasma, and God. However, the idea that there are tiny creatures that can produce illness has been around for a long time. The Roman writer Varro said in the first century BC 'minute animals, invisible to the eye, carried by the air, reach the inside of the body through the mouth, and cause disease'. We know that people in the Middle Ages were aware that disease could be spread from one person to another by the way lepers were shunned. In the 17th century a Dutch shopkeeper, Anthony van Leeuwenhoek, made microscopes that magnified up to 300 times. He was able to see micro-organisms but nobody suggested that these were the cause of disease.

For hundreds of years little progress was made because nobody knew that these germs caused disease and so nobody looked for a way to kill them.

By 1800 there were two main theories about how disease was spread. In some ways they were similar – but they were both wrong.

- **Miasma.** People believed that disease was caused by gases given off by rotting flesh or vegetables. You could tell the gases were present by the smell.

- **Spontaneous generation.** People believed that germs arose from rotting matter. They saw bacteria in rotten meat and assumed that the rotten meat had produced them.

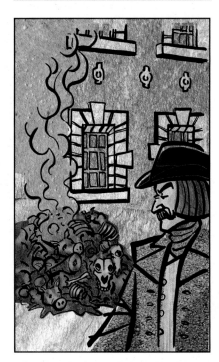

Miasma

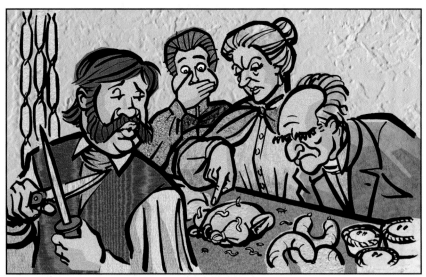

Spontaneous generation

Progress over the next 100 years was rapid. By 1900 people knew that germs caused disease, they knew which germs caused particular diseases, they had developed vaccines to protect people against some diseases, and even drugs to cure people of diseases. The story of how this was done in just 100 years is an amazing one.

Jenner and smallpox vaccination – a great man?

Smallpox

From the late 17th century onwards smallpox killed hundreds of thousands of people. In the 18th century smallpox killed more European children than any other disease.

The first symptoms were a fever and pains in the head, back and muscles. After a few days a rash appeared. The pimples then developed into pustules. If the person survived the disease these pustules dried and the scabs fell off, leaving pockmarks for life.

Smallpox scars were a common sight in the 18th century. It was spread either by the pus from an infected person or by an infected person breathing the virus over someone else. There was no known cure. Instead, ways had to be found of protecting people from it.

The first inoculations

In parts of Africa and China people had for a long time used a primitive sort of inoculation. They scratched pus from the pustules of infected people into their skin. This gave them a mild form of smallpox but most people recovered and did not catch smallpox again. Although people at the time did not realise it, catching the disease had allowed their bodies to develop antibodies against future attacks. They were now protected against the disease.

We know that his method was being used in Constantinople around 1700. In 1717 Lady Mary Wortley Montagu, wife of the British Ambassador in Constantinople, wrote an account of inoculation (Source B).

Lady Mary returned to England at the time of a smallpox epidemic in 1721. She had her five-year-old daughter inoculated in the presence of several important doctors. They were impressed and as news spread even King George I had his grandchildren inoculated.

However, there were problems with inoculation.

- Sometimes it gave people a strong, instead of a mild, attack of smallpox, killing them. Between two and three people in every hundred died from inoculation. (But this has to be compared with the one in five who died from catching the disease naturally.)

- Although it protected the individual who had been inoculated, it did not prevent that person spreading the disease to others.

- Inoculators charged a lot, and so only the rich could benefit.

Despite these problems, inoculators sprang up all over the country. Robert Sutton and his son Daniel were among the best-known inoculators. They improved the method by only taking pus from those with the mildest form of the disease, and by using 'airing houses' where patients were kept until danger of spreading the infection had passed. Daniel inoculated nearly 14,000 people in 1763–4. Charging as much as £20 a patient, he made a fortune. Of course, only the rich could afford this.

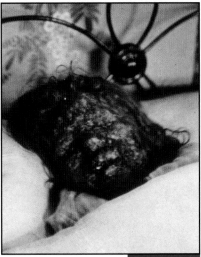

Source A

A photograph of a victim of smallpox in Gloucester in 1896.

The old woman comes with a nutshell full of the matter of the best sort of smallpox, and asks what veins you please to have opened. She immediately rips open that you offer to her with a large needle, and puts into the vein as much venom as can lie upon the head of her needle, and after binds up the little wound with a hollow bit of shell. The young patients are in perfect health to the eighth day. Then the fever begins to seize them, and they keep to their beds two days, very seldom three. Every year thousands undergo this operation. I am very well satisfied of the safety of this experiment, since I intend to try it on my dear little son.

Source B

QUESTIONS

1 What were the disadvantages of inoculation? How did the Suttons try to overcome these?

Biography

Edward Jenner was born in the village of Berkeley in Gloucestershire in 1749. When he was 13 years old he was apprenticed to a surgeon for six years. In 1770 he went to study in London with John Hunter, the greatest surgeon of his time. Hunter encouraged his students not to believe everything in text books but to use their powers of observation and to carry out experiments to test ideas. This would prove useful to Jenner later in his career. Two years later, he returned to Berkeley and set himself up as a country doctor. However, he was not your average country doctor. He kept in touch with John Hunter and continued to conduct experiments.

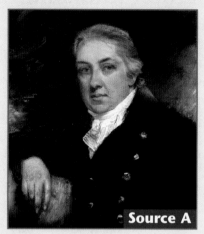

Source A

It was when he was an apprentice that Jenner had first heard that milkers who caught cowpox seemed to be protected from smallpox. He had discussed this with Hunter when he was in London and spent 20 years observing and thinking about it before deciding in 1796 to carry out an experiment. He used a boy called James Phipps who came from a poor local family.

Jenner's description of his experiment, published in 1798. He had to publish this account himself. The Royal Society refused to publish it because of opposition to Jenner's ideas. Jenner waited before publishing the above account because he wanted to carry out more experiments. By the time he published he had vaccinated 23 people.

I selected a healthy boy, about eight years old. The cowpox matter was taken from a sore on the hand of a dairymaid, who was infected by her master's cows, and it was inserted on the 14th May, 1796, into the arm of the boy by means of two superficial incisions, each about an inch long.

On the seventh day he complained of uneasiness in the armpit and on the ninth he became a little chilly, lost his appetite, and had a slight headache. On the day following he was perfectly well.

In order to see whether the boy was secure from the contagion of the smallpox, he was inoculated on the 1st July with matter taken from a smallpox pustule. No disease followed. Several months afterwards he was again inoculated, but there was no illness.

Source B

Vaccination

(The word comes from *vacca* – Latin for cow.)

For centuries there had been a folk tradition that dairymaids and cowhands never caught smallpox. They did catch cowpox (a similar, but much milder version of smallpox) from cows and this seemed to give them protection against smallpox. Some people deliberately gave themselves cowpox. We know that during a smallpox outbreak in 1774, a farmer called Benjamin Jesty took his wife and children to a neighbouring farm in Dorset where the cows had cowpox. He scratched their arms with a needle and rubbed in pus from the pustules on the cows' udders. None of them caught smallpox. This kind of thing was probably going on all over the country. However, it took the genius of Edward Jenner to realise the importance of these methods.

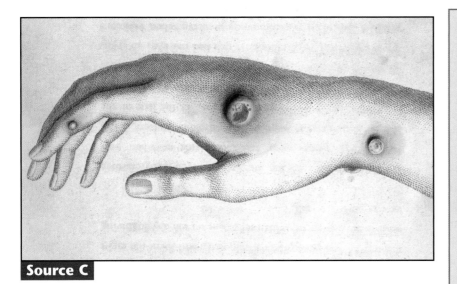

Source C

A dairy maid's hand infected with cowpox (from Jenner's account of his experiment).

Although not everyone accepted vaccination, by 1801 more than 100,000 people had been vaccinated in England. It soon became available in other countries – by 1811 more than 1.7 million people had been vaccinated in France. In 1802 the House of Commons voted to give Jenner £10,000 for his work against smallpox (worth over £2 million today).

Jenner was never to understand how vaccination worked. This was because he did not know that germs cause disease.

The cowpox virus is very similar to the smallpox virus but it is less dangerous and cannot kill or permanently scar people.

When the cowpox virus enters the body, the body creates antibodies to fight it.

When the person comes into contact with the smallpox virus, the antibodies are still in the body and can kill the smallpox virus because it is so similar to the cowpox virus.

Vaccination was much safer than inoculation because it was dangerous to give people even a mild form of smallpox.

Compulsory vaccination

Acceptance of vaccination in England was slow, especially among the poor. In the smallpox epidemic of 1837–40, 35,000 people, mostly children, died. Many had been inoculated, not vaccinated, and so the government made inoculation illegal. In 1853 vaccination for infants became compulsory but there was no way of enforcing it and only about half the children of England and Wales were vaccinated. In 1871 fines or even imprisonment were introduced for parents refusing to have their children vaccinated. Some opposition continued until the end of the century. By 1900 the number of smallpox deaths was almost nil, and in 1909 vaccination stopped being compulsory.

In 1980 the World Health Organisation announced that there had been no cases anywhere in the world for the previous two years. This followed mass vaccination campaigns in countries all round the world. The only place where the smallpox virus now exists is in scientists' laboratories!

And yet, there was much opposition to vaccination throughout the 19th century. Why?

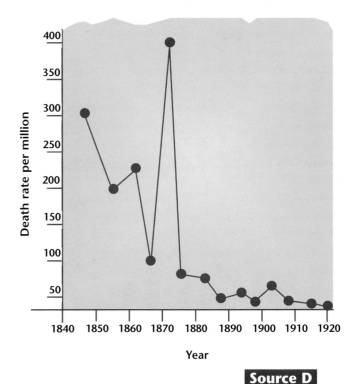

Source D

Deaths from smallpox in England and Wales 1848–1920.

Opposition to vaccination

Although vaccination was much safer than inoculation, there were many people who opposed it:

- Inoculators attacked vaccination because it threatened their livelihoods. They would be put out of work.

- Jenner was not a fashionable London doctor with a big reputation. This turned many London doctors against him. Remember the Royal Society refused to published his findings.

- Clergy preached that it was against God's will to transfer an animal disease to humans. One clergyman claimed vaccination imposed the 'mark of the beast', and was 'against nature'.

- Other clergy claimed that smallpox was a punishment by God for leading an immoral life. The only cure was to lead a pure life.

- Other people had a distaste for taking matter from a sick cow. They said that vaccination introduced a beast's disease into humans whereas inoculation used a human disease. Some were worried that other diseases might be transmitted from the cattle to humans.

- Sometimes vaccination did not work because people did not use it as carefully as Jenner. The vaccine was contaminated sometimes or the needle was not clean. Some doctors mixed the vaccination with water, sometimes dirty, to make it go further. This meant it was too weak to be effective and could even pass on other infections. Many people thought that vaccination spread syphilis. In the 1880s even the government agreed with these claims.

- Many vaccinators were not trained or qualified. They often had to carry out the procedure several times before it worked. Some cut too deeply into the skin, making the child bleed a lot. This simply carried away the cowpox matter. Vaccinators were paid according to the number of successful vaccinations they had carried out, so they did them in a hurry and claimed all were successful even when they were not.

- Jenner was not able to explain how his vaccination worked. This made it difficult for other people to accept vaccination.

- Many people opposed compulsory vaccination. They saw it as the government interfering in what they saw as a family concern. The government had no right to interfere with their children. The Anti-Vaccination League was set up in 1866. In 1871, when fines were introduced, some argued this was unfair on the poor because the rich could afford to pay the fine but the poor went to prison

- Most of the opposition came from the poor – they especially disliked compulsion. They continued to use old methods like inoculation, 'roasting' patients in front of enormous fires, and making children share the same bed to keep each other warm. One doctor wrote 'It is a common sight to see two or three children lying in the same bed with such a load of pustules that their skins stick together.' The poor resented their superiors (the middle classes like doctors) interfering with the working-class way of life while inoculation by a local wise woman was something shared by the community and not imposed by the state.

- The main worry of the poor was to keep their families fed. They did not have time to worry about vaccination. By 1893 33 per cent of infants in London were still not vaccinated.

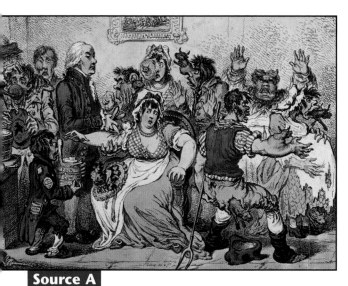

Source A

'The cow-pock – the wonderful effects of the new inoculation.' A cartoon from 1808.

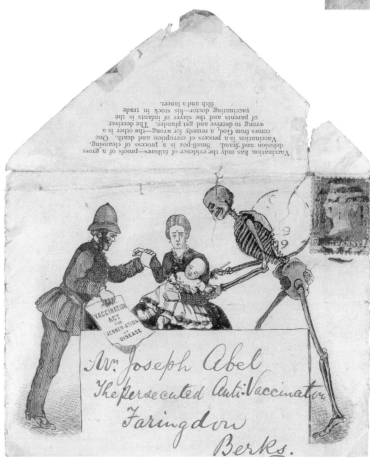

Source B

Anti-vaccination propaganda, 1899. You need to read the back of the envelope.

The text on the back of the envelope reads:

Vaccination has only the evidence of failures—proofs of a gross delusion and fraud. Small-pox is a process of cleansing. Vaccination is a process of corruption and death. One comes from God, a remedy for wrong—the other is a wrong to deceive and get plunder. The deceiver of parents and the slayer of infants is the vaccinating doctor—his stock in trade filth and a lancet.

QUESTIONS

1 Study Sources A and B. Explain why each one was published.

2 Inoculation and even vaccination existed before Jenner. Does this mean he is not important?

3 Imagine you are living in the 1880s. Design a poster to persuade people that vaccination is wrong.

How important was Jenner?

The case *for* Jenner

A form of vaccination had been used by country people for a long time but Jenner was the person who realised how important it might be. He tested it and he published an account of his work, which meant it was accepted by scientists and doctors. Because of Jenner vaccination became widespread and eventually led to the eradication of smallpox and to vaccines for other diseases being developed. Millions of lives have been saved. The country folk who had been using vaccination for years did not do any of this. Was it chance? Not really. It wasn't chance that Jenner came across the idea – it was already widespread and well known. It certainly wasn't chance that Jenner decided to test it scientifically. It was Jenner's genius to realise there was something worth investigating and experimenting with.

The case *against* Jenner

Jenner did not discover anything new. Many people already used vaccination. Jenner stumbled across it. He never understood how it actually worked. It is not even clear that vaccination led to the fall in the number of people dying from smallpox. Many people did not have their children vaccinated and yet the death rate fell. Some historians claim this was because of other factors such as improved living conditions and better diet. People were healthier and so were less likely to catch the disease. Smallpox vaccination was a dead end. Jenner could not explain how vaccination worked and this meant it was impossible for vaccines for other diseases to be developed. It needed the genius of Pasteur to make this happen.

Louis Pasteur and the germ theory of disease

The next important person in this story is Louis Pasteur – he was to open the way for modern medicine to begin by:

- Proving that germs cause disease
- Explaining how vaccination works.

As you read this section you should keep a list of examples of the following factors that helped Pasteur to make his discoveries:

- The needs of French industry
- War
- Rivalry with other scientists
- Pasteur's genius
- Team work
- Chance.

1863 Pasteur develops pasteurisation

By now Pasteur had became a sort of industrial trouble shooter. In 1863 the Emperor asked Pasteur to help the wine industry – France's most important industry and a symbol of France's greatness. Much of the wine was going bad. Pasteur examined the wine under his microscope and announced that there were bacteria in the wine. He showed that these could be killed by heating the wine gently. France's wine industry (worth 500 million Francs a year) was saved. Pasteur then used the same technique with beer and milk. This was a big step forward in making liquids safe from germs and safe for people to drink.

1857 Germs make liquids go sour

Pasteur was born in France in 1822. He studied chemistry at first but was soon investigating the links between chemistry and biology. He became Dean of Science at the University of Lille in 1854. Lille was a manufacturing centre for alcohol but the manufacturers were having great problems – their production of beetroot alcohol was disappointingly low because the liquid was going sour. Something was going wrong with the process of fermentation. One of the manufacturers, Monsieur Bigo, came to Pasteur for help. Pasteur examined the juice under a microscope and saw thousands of micro-organisms. He realised that where the liquid was going sour, the micro-organisms were a different shape.

- He concluded that the micro-organisms were making the liquid go sour.
- He then studied milk and wine and concluded that microbes were also responsible for making them go sour.

1864 Proving spontaneous generation wrong and the germ theory right

During his work on wine Pasteur had become convinced that germs were causing liquids to go sour and that the germs were coming from the air around us. This meant he was now locked in a battle with the great defender of spontaneous generation, Felix Pouchet. Pasteur loved turning science into a battlefield, he loved an argument. In 1857 he moved to Paris and over the next few years conducted a series of experiments to prove he was right. Pasteur received important help from the Emperor Louis Napoleon. His government gave Pasteur research assistants and money to pay for a new laboratory. The Emperor thought that Pasteur's discoveries were adding to France's reputation. The most famous of Pasteur's experiments involved the use of swan-necked flasks.

Pasteur used swan-necked flasks with long necks and openings that were only one millimetre wide (see Source B). He boiled the liquid in some of the flasks but left the liquid in the others unboiled. After 24 hours the liquid in the unboiled flasks was covered by mould, while the boiled liquid was not. He then snapped off the necks of these flasks and soon mould was growing on the liquid. Pasteur claimed that the long, narrow necks of the flasks had captured the germs that entered with the air. When the necks were broken and the air could get through, germs carried by the air could reach the liquid.

In 1864 Pasteur repeated some of his experiments in front of France's leading scientists. He was a great showman. He loved doing his experiments in public. In fact, he was a show-off and he completely humiliated Pouchet as Source C shows. Most of his fellow scientists were convinced. One of them announced 'spontaneous generation is no more, M. Pasteur has resolved the question'.

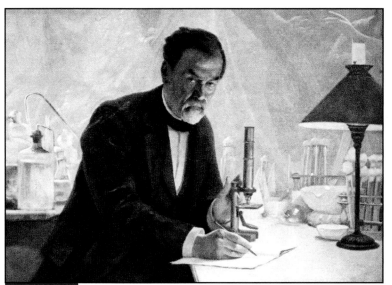

Source A

Pasteur in his
laboratory.

1865 Pasteur shows that disease in animals is caused by germs

So far Pasteur had not investigated any animal diseases. However, in 1865 this changed. An epidemic was destroying the French silkworm industry and Pasteur was called in to help. Millions of francs were at stake. Pasteur discovered that the silkworms were dying of a disease called pebrine and he showed that the disease was being spread by a living organism in the air.

A swan-necked flask as used by
Pasteur.

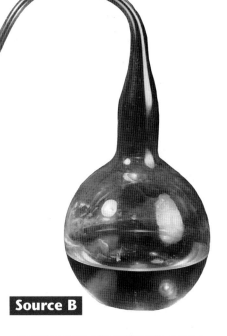

Source B

1865 Pasteur turns to human disease but suffers setbacks

A personal tragedy suddenly turned his attention to humans and the threat disease posed to them. Camille, Pasteur's two-year-old daughter, died. By now Pasteur was convinced that the microbes he had discovered in the air were the cause of human diseases – but he had to prove it. His daughter's death made him decide that this was what he must now do. Only a few weeks later Pasteur started work on human disease.

However, personal tragedy was not his only motivation. In 1867, when trying to persuade the government to pay for a new laboratory for the investigation of infectious disease, he argued this was needed because of 'the necessity of maintaining the scientific superiority of France against the efforts of rival nations'.

In 1865 Paris was hit by cholera. This was Pasteur's chance to prove the germ theory. He squatted by the ventilators leading from a hospital cholera ward, taking samples from the air. When he examined them under a microscope all he could see were lots of different organisms. He had no idea which was the one causing cholera. Pasteur was stuck! Three years later he suffered another setback when he had a stroke that paralysed the left side of his body.

And therefore, gentlemen, I have taken my drop of water. But it is dead. It is dead because I have kept it from the only thing man cannot produce, from the germs which float in the air, from Life, for Life is a germ and a germ is Life. Never will the theory of spontaneous generation recover from the mortal blow of this simple experiment.

Source C

Pasteur speaking in his lecture
of 1864.

The Great Rivals

The next part of the story involves a scientist from Germany – Robert Koch. He was similar to Pasteur in many ways – ambitious, quarrelsome and always happy to rub his rivals' noses in the dust by defeating them in argument.

Pasteur and Koch became great personal rivals. This rivalry was increased because France and Germany were also rivals at the time. In 1870–71 they fought in a war which Germany won. Koch served in the war as a doctor with the German army. This defeat made Pasteur hate Germany. The two men now competed with each other for personal glory but also for the glory of their own nation. This rivalry drove both men on to make a series of astounding advances in the period 1873 to 1885.

Pasteur (France)

1879 – shows how anthrax infects animals

Pasteur began working again. He showed that when sheep dying of anthrax were buried they were contaminating the soil. Earthworms were carrying the disease to the surface and infecting more animals. Farmers began to burn the animals instead which helped stop the spread of anthrax.

1879 – shows germs carried by nurses causing infection in hospitals

Pasteur was now spending as much time in hospitals as in laboratories. His motto was 'Seek the microbe'. There had been an epidemic of puerperal fever in maternity hospitals. Pasteur proved 'It is the nursing and medical staff who carry the microbe from an infected woman to a healthy one' and he showed that it was the streptococcus microbe that was doing the damage.

1880 – shows how vaccination works

Pasteur had realised that he could make faster progress if he put a research team together. Pasteur was a chemist and needed people working with him who knew more about medicine. Two of the people he employed were Emile Roux and Charles Chamberland, both young doctors. They started to study chicken cholera which was destroying flocks of chickens. The farmers were losing a lot of money. Pasteur was sent the head of a chicken which had died. He quickly found the microbe that caused the disease and was able to grow more.

Over the summer of 1880 he left Chamberland with instructions to inoculate some chickens with the germs. For some reason Chamberland forgot to do it – perhaps he was in a rush to get off on his holidays. He left the germs on a shelf. The laboratory then closed for the summer. When Chamberland returned he carried out the inoculations. The chickens became ill but to everyone's surprise they then recovered. They should have died. Chamberland had stumbled across a great discovery but he did not realise it. It took Pasteur's genius to work out what had happened. He had studied Jenner's work on vaccination very carefully and this gave him an idea. He ordered that a new batch of the germs be made and the same chickens be injected with it. The chickens survived again. He then had some new chickens injected – they died. Pasteur's guess was right – the germs that Chamberland had left over the summer had become weakened through being exposed to the air. When injected into the chickens these weakened germs had somehow given the chickens protection from the disease. Was Pasteur lucky? No! As he said 'chance only favours prepared minds'.

Koch (Germany)

1873 – makes it easier to study germs

Koch began as a doctor but in 1873 he became District Medical Officer in the town of Wollstein. This gave him time for research. The farms around him were suffering from the disease of anthrax and this is what he decided to research. He found a way of looking at micro-organisms through a microscope while protecting them from infection from the air. He did this by making a small trough in a glass slide where the infected substance went. This was covered with a second slide. All the edges of both slides were then sealed.

1876 – discovers the germ causing anthrax

For the first time it was shown that a specific germ caused a specific disease. Koch fed the germ with fluid from an ox's eye and watched it grow. He then injected it into mice and when it killed them he knew he had found proof that there were different types of germs and each type caused a different disease. He had proved the central point in Pasteur's germ theory.

1879 – stains and photographs germs, and develops a method for showing which germ causes a particular disease

Koch was worried that Pasteur was getting all the credit for his work. He began to develop ways of staining micro-organisms with dyes – this made it easier to identify and study them. He used the new Zeiss lens to see and photograph tiny bacteria whose presence had not previously been known e.g. the bacteria that cause septicaemia (a disease often caught by patients who had had surgery).

He also found a way of proving which germ caused a particular disease. He injected a mixture of bacteria into an animal. When the animal became ill with a disease, he took blood from the animal and injected another with the blood. Because the bacteria causing the disease grew most rapidly, by the time this was repeated with several animals only one type of bacteria remained – the one causing the disease.

Once Koch found a way of identifying different germs, others were quickly discovered.

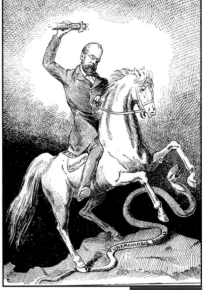

Source A

A cartoon showing Koch.

1882	Typhoid
1883	Cholera
1884	Tetanus
1886	Pneumonia
1894	Plague
1949	Polio virus

Source B

Once Koch found a way of identifying different germs, others were quickly discovered.

1880 – develops a way of growing germs

Koch then made an enormous step forward in the study of germs – he showed how to grow pure cultures of bacteria on potato. This made them much easier to study than in a quivering drop of liquid. He then found an even better method – by suspending the bacteria in solid agar-jelly.

1881-82 – develops a vaccine for anthrax

Pasteur had begun to understand how vaccines worked. (He used the word vaccination in honour of Jenner.) He was sure that vaccines could be developed for other diseases. By 1881 he had produced a weakened form of the anthrax germ and was using it successfully with rabbits and sheep. He then received the kind of challenge he could not resist – to carry out a public test of his anthrax vaccine. The test was arranged for May 1882. On 5 May farmers, doctors, scientists and journalists flocked to the farm. The diary entries above right show the method Pasteur used to prove his vaccine. He was triumphant. He had now found two vaccines. Journalists made sure that he was now famous all over Europe.

Pasteur (France)

5th May
25 sheep injected with anthrax vaccine. Another 25 sheep not injected.

31st May
Both lots of sheep injected with anthrax.

2nd June
The first 25 sheep all healthy. The second 25 sheep all dead.

1885 – discovers a vaccine for rabies

Jolted by Koch's success with tuberculosis, Pasteur turned his attention to human diseases. He was trying to find a vaccine for rabies. In 1885 he tested his vaccine on a boy, Joseph Meister, who had been bitten by a rabid dog. If nothing was done the boy would certainly die. Pasteur knew his vaccine had worked on dogs. He also knew that rabies develops slowly in humans. There might be time to save the boy. Joseph was given 13 injections over 14 days and he was saved. Pasteur had used a vaccine on a human and it had worked. This led to other vaccines being discovered.

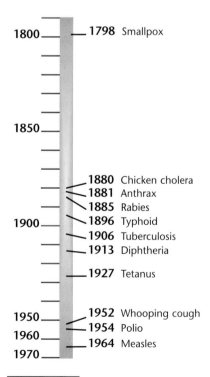

1800	1798 Smallpox
1850	
	1880 Chicken cholera
	1881 Anthrax
	1885 Rabies
1900	1896 Typhoid
	1906 Tuberculosis
	1913 Diphtheria
	1927 Tetanus
1950	1952 Whooping cough
1960	1954 Polio
	1964 Measles
1970	

Source B

Once Pasteur had worked out how vaccination worked, others were quickly discovered.

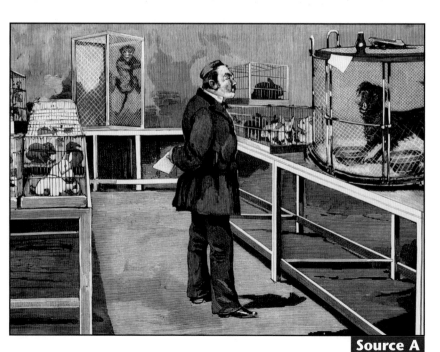

Source A

Pasteur in his laboratory during his work on rabies.

Koch (Germany)

1881–82 – discovers the germ causing tuberculosis

Koch received the news of Pasteur's anthrax vaccine with gloom. He believed Pasteur had stolen much of his work on anthrax. He decided that his next work would be done in secret until he was ready to report all his results. Could he be the first to discover the germ that caused a human disease? He chose tuberculosis, a disease that killed millions.The tuberculosis germ is extremely small and for this reason had been missed by scientists. Koch found a way of staining the microbe so that it stood out against the surrounding tissue. He then grew the germ and injected it into healthy animals. When they died he knew he had found the cause of a human disease.

This was a major breakthrough. His own pupils were able to discover the germs causing other diseases. This would then lead to the development of vaccines to prevent the diseases, and to drugs to cure people of the diseases.

QUESTIONS

1 Pasteur and Koch are both very important in the history of medicine. Make a list of the main discoveries of each. Choose the ten most important developments. Plot these developments on a grid with dates along the bottom from 1857 to 1885. Use different colours for Pasteur's and Koch's discoveries.

2 Choose the two developments which you think were the most important and explain why.

3 Look at the factors listed on page 112. Using the work of Pasteur and Koch find an example of each factor helping progress.

EXAM PRACTICE QUESTIONS

(a) Explain the theory of spontaneous generation.

(b) Explain how Pasteur proved the theory of spontaneous generation was wrong.

(c) 'Koch's work was more important than Pasteur's.' Explain how far you agree with this statement.

The search for cures

Chemical drugs

The next step was to find cures for diseases. Paul Ehrlich worked with Koch but then ran his own research institute. On the day it opened in 1906 he gave a speech announcing what work his institute would do. He believed it was possible to find chemical substances that would cure diseases – he called them magic bullets. They would seek out and destroy the microbes causing a particular disease in the human body without harming the body. He believed that for every microbe causing disease it would be possible to develop a chemical that fitted the microbe like a key does a lock.

One of the diseases he tried to find a cure for was syphilis – a sexually transmitted disease that could lead to insanity, paralysis, heart failure and blindness. It also caused disfigurement – faces rotting away with ulcers. Only one in five people suffering from the disease in France recovered. Ten per cent of all deaths were due to it!

Ehrlich and his assistants tried hundreds of different chemical compounds without success. Then, in 1909 a Japanese scientist, Dr Hata, joined the institute. He re-tested some of the compounds and found that No. 606 worked. Salverson 606 was the first chemical to seek out and destroy a microbe within the human body. But it was effective only on the syphilis germ.

Over the next 20 years scientists tried to find other chemical compounds. They had no success until the 1930s when a German scientist found that Prontosil, a red dye, worked against the germs which caused sepsis and blood poisoning. In 1935 he tried it out on his own daughter who was dying from blood poisoning and it saved her. Scientists discovered that it was the sulphonamide chemical in the dye that was killing the germs (sulphonamide means chemicals made from coal tar). This led to a number of sulphonamide drugs being produced for diseases such as pneumonia and meningitis. By 1941, 1700 tons of 'sulpha drugs' were prescribed by doctors to 10 million Americans.

Natural drugs – Penicillin, the first antibiotic

Staphylococcus germs remained undefeated. They protected themselves by producing a substance that weakened the effect of the magic bullets. However, an answer had already been found, not in drugs made from chemicals but in a naturally growing mould.

Fungi had often been used in popular medicine for treating wounds and Pasteur himself had noticed that some kinds of bacteria killed other bacteria. This led to the idea that bacteria could be used to kill bacteria – what later would be called antibiotics. The first and most important antibiotic was penicillin. Study Part 1 of the story of its discovery and answer the question that follows it.

CASE STUDY

How important was Fleming in the development of Penicillin?

As you are reading through the story of penicillin make notes on how the following factors helped or hindered progress: chance, individual brilliance, war, government, industry.

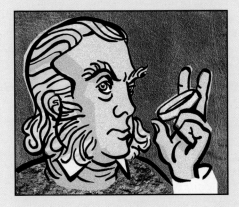

Part 1 – The discovery of penicillin

In 1872 Lister noticed that penicillin mould killed bacteria and in 1884 he used it to successfully treat an infected wound of a nurse. But he made no notes and took it no further.

Alexander Fleming, a bacteriologist at St Mary's Hospital in London was sent to France during the First World War to study the treatment of wounds of soldiers infected by streptococci and staphylococci germs. He found that chemical antiseptics were not working on deeply infected wounds. The suffering of the soldiers from their dreadful wounds greatly affected Fleming. He became determined to find a better way of treating infected wounds after the war had ended.

In 1928 Fleming was working on staphylococci germs. When he went on holiday he left a pile of culture plates on his bench. When he returned he was sorting out the plates when he noticed a large blob of mould on one of the plates. Around this mould the staphyloccal germs had gone. He said to himself 'that's funny' and took a sample of the mould. (It seems that spores from a mould grown by a colleague in room directly above Fleming had floated down into his laboratory.)

Fleming seems to have realised that he had made an important discovery because he kept the plate and mould and showed them to his colleagues, but nobody was interested.

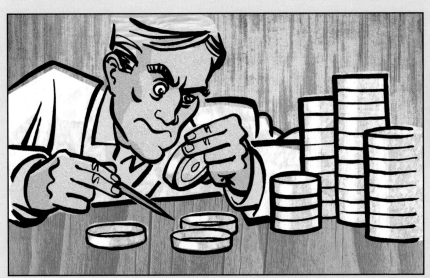

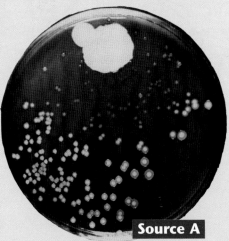

Source A

A photograph of the original dish showing the effect of penicillin.

CASE STUDY

Fleming carried out some experiments on the mould. He grew more of it, produced juice from it, and began to draw up a list of all the germs that it killed. He then used it on living cells and found that when it was diluted it did no harm to the living cells but still killed bacteria. It looked as though he had found a natural antiseptic that would kill germs but not harm the body.

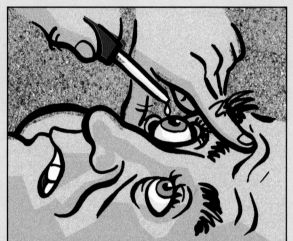

Fleming then tested penicillin on rabbits and found that when mixed with blood it lost a lot of its strength. It also took over four hours to act against germs – perhaps it would not be useful after all.

Fleming used penicillin as a local antiseptic on a scientist's eye that had conjunctivitis. The infection cleared up, but when he used it in deep wounds it didn't work. It also took a long time to produce enough penicillin to treat just one person.

In 1929 Fleming wrote up all his findings into a paper – one of the most important medical papers ever written and one that has affected the lives of almost every human being on earth. However, at the time nobody recognised its importance. This was probably Fleming's own fault – he had not tried injecting penicillin into infected animals, he had only used it as a local antiseptic. This meant he had not provided the evidence that it was an important breakthrough.

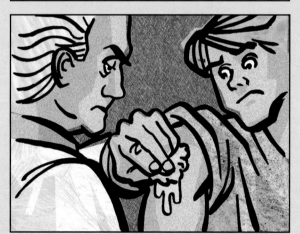

It is important to note what Fleming wrote at this time: 'Penicillin may be an efficient antiseptic for application to, or injection into, areas infected with penicillin-sensitive microbes. It is quite likely that penicillin will be used in the treatment of septic wounds.'

During the 1930s Fleming used penicillin as a local antiseptic a few times but gradually lost interest in it.

Q1 Some books make the following claims. Test each one against what you have just read. Are they right?
(a) The discovery of penicillin was a complete accident. Fleming was very lucky – it could have happened to anyone.
(b) Fleming did not realise the importance of penicillin.
(c) Fleming was to blame for the fact that nobody else realised how important penicillin was.

Part 2 – The development of penicillin

In 1938 two Oxford University scientists, Howard Florey and Ernst Chain, were working on natural substances that would kill germs. They read Fleming's paper and started to work on penicillin. They gradually got more and more excited about what they found and in 1939 they applied for a government grant. They received only £25! The government was more interested in the war effort (the Second World War started in 1939) and it did not see that penicillin could help win the war. The £25 was nowhere near enough to pay for the wages of research assistants and equipment and so Florey turned to America and received grants for five years.

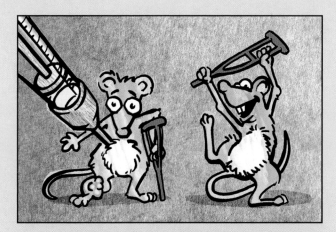

Chain used freeze drying to extract pure penicillin. He found that penicillin was destroyed in the stomach so it was no good giving it by mouth. However, infected mice that were injected with penicillin recovered. (Remember that Fleming had not tried injecting penicillin into animals.)

The next move was to test penicillin on humans. For this Florey and Chain needed 3,000 times the dose – and it took a long time to produce even small amounts of the juice. Florey approached pharmaceutical firms such as Wellcome but they were not interested because there was no proof it would work on humans. Besides they were too busy producing other medicines for the war. It seemed as though the demands of war would kill off further work on penicillin.

So Florey decided to turn his university department into a factory to produce penicillin. The mould was grown in hundreds of hospital bedpans. The juice then had to be slowly extracted. By the beginning of 1941 there was enough penicillin juice to use on one human.

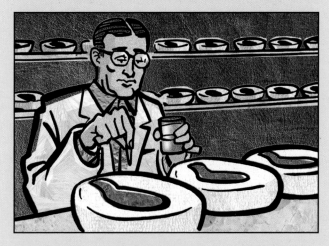

Albert Alexander, a 43-year-old policeman, had been scratched by a rosebush. Staphylococci germs had invaded the wound and infected his whole body. One of his eyes had already been removed. Sulphonamides had been useless. When he was injected with penicillin the swellings started to go down but the treatment had to stop after five days because there was no penicillin left. The infection took hold again and he died. However, other patients were cured when penicillin was used.

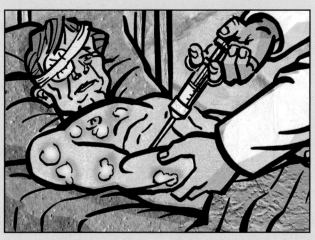

CASE STUDY

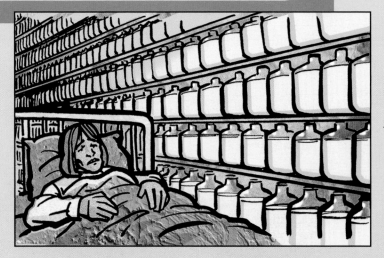

The main problem was still that they could not grow penicillin fast enough. They needed much more of it (it took 2,000 litres to treat one case of sepsis). Florey went to America to look for help, just at the right time. In November 1941 Japan had attacked Pearl Harbor and this had drawn America into the war. The American government realised that the production of penicillin could be of vital importance for American troops. It agreed to fund several chemical companies to mass produce penicillin in enormous vats holding tens of thousands of gallons of the liquid.

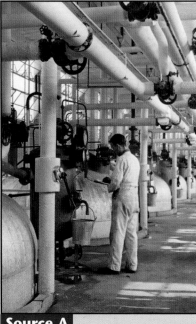

Source A

Huge fermentation tanks used in the production of penicillin.

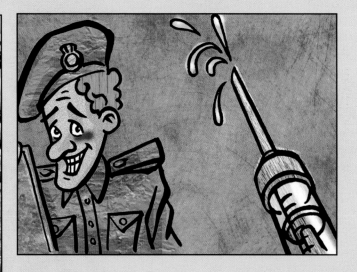

By June 1943, 425 million units of penicillin were being produced each month – enough for 170 patients. By June 1944 this had risen to 100,000 million a month – enough for 40,000 cases. By the end of the war a quarter of a million soldiers were being treated. Drug companies in Britain were producing a fraction of this although it was still used to treat thousands of British soldiers with gonorrhoea in North Africa and get them back to fighting.

Lieutenant Colonel Pulvertaft's description of the first use of penicillin during the war – in North Africa in 1943.

Source B

We had enormous numbers of infected wounded, terrible burn cases among crews of the armoured cars, and fractures infected with streptococci. The medical journals told us that the sulphonamides would get the better of any infection. My own experience was that they had absolutely no effect on these cases. The last thing I tried was penicillin, I had very little of it. The first man I tried it on was a young New Zealand officer. He had been in bed for six months with compound fractures in both legs. His sheets were saturated with pus. We injected him with a very weak solution of penicillin. I gave three injections a day. In ten days the left leg was cured, and in a month's time the young fellow was back on his feet.

Who should get the credit for penicillin?

The importance of penicillin cannot be over-estimated. It was the first antibiotic drug and today different varieties have been developed. It has saved the lives of millions of people. Unless you are allergic to it (around ten per cent of people are) you have almost certainly been prescribed it by a doctor at some time. It is safe and can be given in large doses. Here are just some of the diseases penicillins are used to treat: chronic bronchitis, gonorrhoea, impetigo, meningitis, pneumonia, septicaemia, septic arthritis, syphilis, tonsillitis, urinary tract infection, wounds, boils, abscesses.

In 1945 Fleming, Florey and Chain were all awarded the Nobel prize for their work on pencillin. However, most people only know Fleming's name. To explain this we have to go back to 1942, during the war, when Fleming came back into the story. A patient of his at St Mary's Hospital was dying from meningitis. It looked as though nothing would save him. Fleming had been following Florey's work and got some penicillin from him. The patient was given some injections and recovered. The papers got hold of the story. Sir Almoth Wright – Fleming's boss at St Mary's – was worried that Fleming, and indeed St Mary's Hospital, were not going to get any credit and so he wrote to *The Times* newspaper.

In the leading article on penicillin in your issue yesterday, you refrained from putting the laurel wreath for this discovery round anyone's brow. I would, with your permission, supplement your article by pointing out that the credit should be given to Professor Alexander Fleming of this research laboratory. For he is the discoverer of penicillin and was the author also of the original suggestion that this substance might prove to have important applications in medicine.

Source C

Reporters now besieged Fleming. They also went to see Florey but he sent them away. So they returned to Fleming and in their reports he was portrayed as the main hero. But who was more important in the story of penicillin, Fleming or Chain and Florey?

EXAM PRACTICE QUESTIONS

(a) Describe how Fleming discovered penicillin.

(b) Did war hinder or help the development of penicillin?

(c) Was the work of Florey and Chain more important than that of Fleming? Explain your answer.

Public health – sewers and cesspits

For the exam you will need to know:

- ☑ The state of towns and the dangers this posed to health

- ☑ Why people did not want governments to improve public health

- ☑ Reasons why public health was improved later in the nineteenth century

- ☑ The reforms of the Liberal Government 1906–14

- ☑ The establishment of the National Health Service.

1700	5.83 million
1750	6.25
1800	9.16
1850	17.92
1900	35.52

Source A

The population of England and Wales 1700-1900.

Between 1700 and 1900 there were two important developments which made the problem of public health a very serious one: there was a population explosion (see Source A); and there was a massive movement of people from the country to towns.

The Industrial Revolution of the 18th and 19th centuries led to factories being developed. People flocked from the countryside to these factories for work. Around the factories enormous towns and cities rapidly grew where people lived in terrible overcrowded conditions. Factory owners or speculators provided houses for the workers as cheaply as they could. They were often badly built and damp, small and squeezed in against each other.

Towns and cities grew far too quickly for proper sewage, drainage and water supplies to be built. This soon led to squalid, over-crowded slums with overflowing cesspools, contaminated water pumps, and polluted air.

In 1847 the town of Reading had 378 pigsties, 2,500 houses and courts, and 17,000 people. But there were no sewers – just open privies. Human waste often lay in the streets for weeks – sometimes farmers collected it for manure or it was used for brick-making. Piped water was available to few - and it was often dirty. Where water pumps were provided people often had to queue for hours because one pump was providing water for thousands. The pumps were usually only turned on for one or two hours a day! Most people used wells or a nearby river. A few bought it from water carriers. Where there were sewers, they ran into the very rivers that people got their water from or led to cesspits that were overflowing and rarely emptied.

Most people thought disease was caused by miasma (bad air) from stagnant water or rotting animals. Some local authorities did try to remove stagnant water and decaying matter, while others like Exeter burned barrels of tar in the streets to get rid of the bad air.

Source B

London housing in the second half of the 19th century

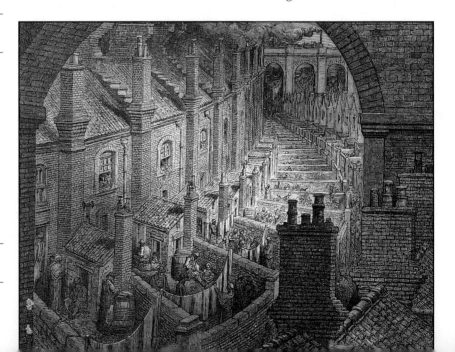

Diphtheria – came to Britain in the 1850s. Spread by droplets from coughing and sneezing, and through contaminated milk.

Typhus – spread by lice which have fed on an infected human. The lice then carry the micro-organism which is spread through the excrement dust of the lice through scratches of human skin, or by breathing it in.

Cholera – spread in drinking water or food contaminated by the faeces of an infected person. It was not a carrier disease so the only solution was adequate sanitation.

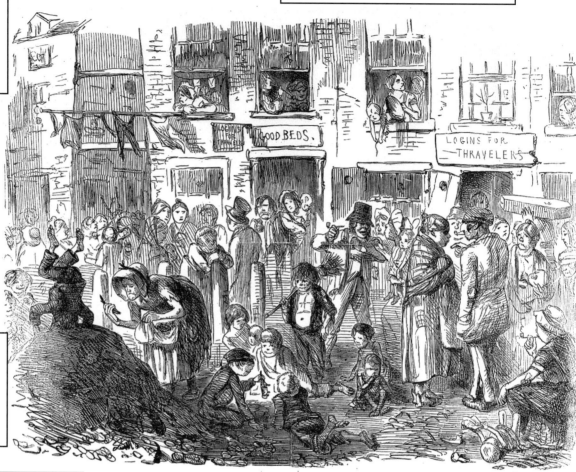

Smallpox – spread by a virus which is present in the nose and throat of the infected person, and in the smallpox blisters on the skin.

Typhoid – spread by fouled water, milk or other foods. An infected person can spread it through the food they touch, or by their excrement fouling the water supply.

Scarlet fever and **measles** – mainly affected children. Spread by droplet infection (coughing and sneezing), but can be carried in clothes, or food. Measles can be spread by touch.

Tuberculosis – the bacteria are spread through spitting, coughing or sneezing, or on contaminated eating utensils, or in contaminated milk and dairy products.

QUESTIONS

1 On pages 124–5 are descriptions and drawings of living conditions in towns in the 19th century and in which diseases were spread. Draw a chart with the diseases listed on the left. For each disease find two examples from pages 124–5 of where it could spread. Enter them on the chart.

Source C

A cartoon called 'A Court for King Cholera' drawn in the middle of the 19th century.

LONDON TODAY

5 May 1851

IS THOMAS CRAPPER WASTING HIS TIME?

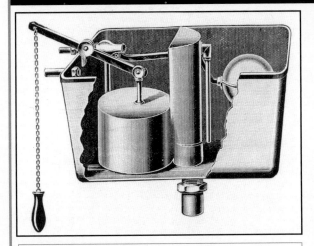

THE FUTURE?
Thomas Crapper's Water Waste Preventer has been installed in Buckingham Palace

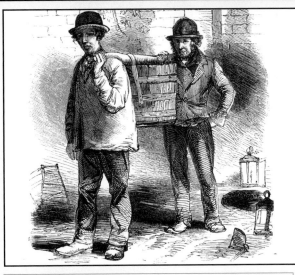

THE PRESENT
The night soil men who empty our cesspits at night

One of the great attractions at the Great Exhibition has been the flushing water closets designed by Thomas Crapper and others. However, many ladies have complained that when they peered down to see how it worked they were presented with a reflection of their own behinds. This had led to a demand that the bowls should be patterned. We ask a more important question – what is the point of a flushing water closet when most houses are not connected to sewers?

THE DISGRACE OF OUR TOWNS – MEDIEVAL CONDITIONS REPORTED

Many people are still living in conditions similar to those in the Middle Ages, reports Harry Scoop, our reporter. His report continues, 'To get to these people you have to penetrate courts reeking with poisonous gases arising from sewage and refuse scattered in all directions. Courts, many of which the sun never penetrates, which are never visited by a breath of fresh air, and which have never seen a drop of fresh water. You have to grope your way along dark and filthy passages swarming with vermin.'

Dung heap keeper found guilty

Mr Gore, a dung heap keeper, was prosecuted for his dung heaps which were 14 feet high – higher than the nearby houses whose value had dropped. In these heaps, witnesses said, were dead animals, decayed potatoes, brewery refuse, and cabbage leaves. The smells were still strong 400 feet away. Gore produced a team of scavengers who claimed they were healthy and never sick. One said that working on the heaps gave him a good appetite. Despite this Mr Gore was found guilty

Four months' hard labour for butcher

Mr Harris, a London butcher, was yesterday sentenced to four months' hard labour for selling bad meat. One witness told the court, 'The pork was covered in pus and decomposed, the veal was green and slimy.' Harris claimed that the meat was only 'muggy' and would be 'alright when it was wiped'.

It has long been a cause for concern that the poor, on the rare occasion they buy meat, buy the cheapest grades. This means they are buying diseased meat. The cheapest meat to buy is bacon with black spots – this means it has anthrax! It is no wonder there is so much disease!

WOMAN POISONED BY THE RIVER THAMES

A woman tried to drown herself in the Thames last Thursday. She was fished out alive but died five days later, poisoned by the water she had swallowed.

Dear Sir

I am appalled by the lack of personal hygiene of many of my patients. I admit many of them are poor, but this should not stop them from keeping clean. Many of them smell of stale urine. I can smell many of my patients approaching my house. When I am treating them I have to keep the door open because of the smell. Many of them only wash the exposed parts of their bodies and work and sleep in the same clothes for weeks.

Yours sincerely

Dr R Liddle

QUESTIONS

1 Compare the living conditions described on these pages with those reported by *London Today* in the Middle Ages on pages 78–9. Have conditions got better, or worse? Give reasons for your answer.

Living in 19th-century towns and cities

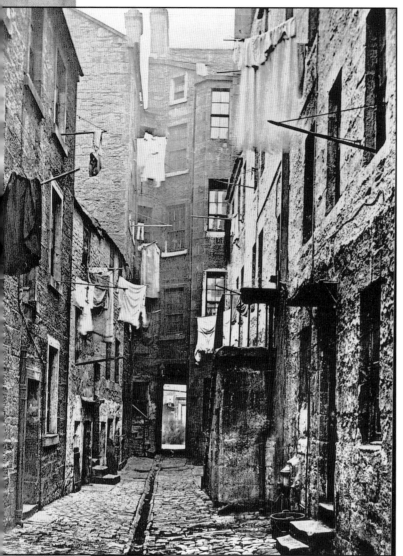

Source A

A photograph of tenements in Glasgow in the 1860s.

One nuisance frequently occurs in these districts. The houses of the poor sometimes surround a court, into which the doors and windows open at the back of the dwelling. Porkers, who feed pigs in the town, often pay a small sum for the rent of the court, which is often covered with pigsties, and converted into a dung-heap and receptacle of the rotting garbage, upon which the animals are fed, and also the refuse which is flung into it from the surrounding dwellings. Slaughter-houses exist in the most narrowest and most filthy streets in the town. The drainage from these houses, deeply tinged with blood and other animal matters, frequently flows down the gutter of the street, and stagnates in the ruts and pools.

Source B

A description of Manchester written in the middle of the 19th century.

In the middle of the road was usually seen the gutter, which carried away the rubbish of the city. But as late as 1808 there was but one water-closet in the city, and that emptied itself into the open street; it was the habit of the people to have tubs within their own houses for the necessary filth, and which towards evening were carried through the streets in order to be emptied into the river. The city depended for its water supply on rain, sunken wells and the river.

Source C

A description of Exeter in 1845.

In one cul-de-sac in Leeds there are 34 houses and in ordinary times, there dwell in these houses 340 persons, or ten to every house. In these houses, brothers and sisters, and lodgers of both sex are found occupying the same sleeping room with the parents. To build the largest number of cottages on the smallest space seems to have been the aim of the builders. The name of this place is Boot and Shoe Yard from whence was removed, in the days of cholera, 75 cartloads of manure which had been untouched for years.

Source D

An account of Leeds in 1842.

Source E

A description of children working in glass manufacturing in the middle of the 19th century.

The hard labour and the intense heat engender in children stunted growth, infections of the eye, bowel complaints, rheumatism and bronchitis. Many of the children are often blind for weeks at a time, suffer from violent nausea, vomiting and coughs. They usually die young of chest infections.

Other dangers to health

- Food presented many dangers e.g. milk was not boiled by mothers to kill germs until the 1880s. Even then many doctors opposed the practice – they claimed it took away the goodness of the milk. However, many cows were diseased; some were tubercular. Milk was made more dangerous when it was watered down, as this was often done with dirty water carrying typhoid germs.

- Food was often adulterated. Harmful substances were added to make food go further and to swindle the customers. Alum was added to bread to whiten it, beer had substances added to it that damaged the nervous system, and children's sweets were coloured with lead carbonate and copper arsenate. Sugar had sand added to it while sawdust was added to flour, and water and animal fats added to butter.

- Working conditions caused much disease – boy chimney sweeps developed cancer from the soot, miners suffered from silicosis and cotton workers from brown lung disease.

- There were few properly trained doctors in poor areas and the poor could not afford them. Most people went without any kind of medical aid.

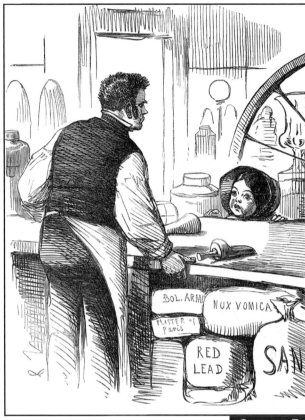

Source F

A cartoon from 1845 showing the different ways food was adulterated.

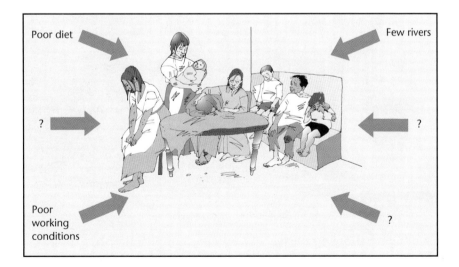

QUESTIONS

1 Copy this diagram and complete it by showing three other causes of poor health.

Why was nothing done?

You have already seen that these terrible conditions were caused by towns and cities growing too quickly. But why was nothing done to improve these conditions and why, when attempts were made to do something, was there opposition?

A lack of understanding

One reason is that people at this time did not understand that germs caused disease. (Remember Pasteur did not prove his germ theory until 1864.) Most people believed disease was spread by miasma – gases given off by rotting flesh and vegetables. This theory did lead some people to demand that towns be cleaned up as you will see later but it also meant that the importance of clean water was not understood.

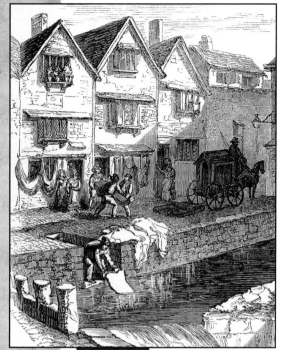

Source A

A drawing of the clothes of cholera victims in Exeter in 1832 being washed in the river from which people got their drinking water.

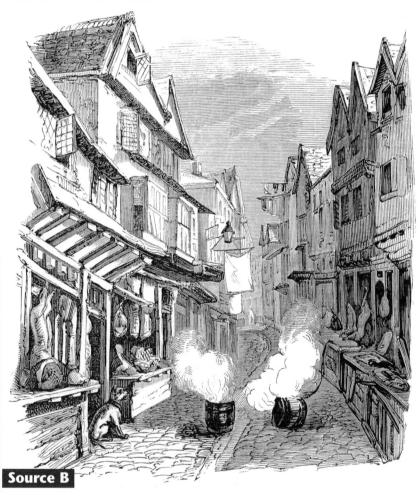

Source B

A drawing showing barrels of tar being burnt in the streets of Exeter in 1832. It was thought that this would stop cholera spreading.

NOTICE!!!

We are credibly informed by a correspondent that the much-admired

JAPANESE CHEROOTS

are highly recommended by the faculty abroad as being a sure preventive of that raging disorder the

Cholera Morbus;

they have been recently imported into this Country, and are found to be of that mild and fragrant nature that they may be used by

The Fair Sex

without producing nausea. Their confirmed anti-contagious virtues and delicate fragrance have already procured them a very high and just estimation.

Vide Morning Herald, Nov. 12, 1831.

ARLISS, Printer, Addle Street, Wood Street, Cheapside.

Source C

An advertisement for cigars, 1831.

QUESTIONS

1 Explain how Sources A, B, and C show why people did not support campaigns for cleaner water.

Attitudes about the poor and the government

Even if germ theory was not yet proved, the miasma theory did lead some people to argue that towns needed cleaning up. There were those who saw that there was a connection between filth and squalor and disease. Why was still nothing done? The answer lies in the attitudes of people at the time. The idea of *laissez-faire* said that it was not the job of the government to keep people healthy. The job of the government was to keep law and order, not to keep people clean. This was because some people believed that:

- People should help themselves, they should not depend on others because this would make them weak. It would lead to them depending on others for everything.

- The cause of disease was poverty. The poor were poor because they were lazy. It was up to them to get a job and get out of poverty.

- If the government interfered and made local councils clean things up this would be a great threat to everyone's freedom. It would give too much power to the government.

- It would cost a lot of money to pay for a clean water supply and proper drains and sewers. The middle-class ratepayers knew they would have to pay for it all. They did not want to do this because many of the benefits would go to the poor who did not pay rates and did not deserve better conditions.

> In 1841 the Exeter Water Company laid four inch pipes along the three streets of St Thomas. The pipe is fixed by the Company. The water is always on. The annual charge for the poorest house is 5s. The company entered St Thomas with the expectation that the demand would be great. It has been trifling. They supply only 47 families. This is only 5 per cent of the population, and only 1 per cent of the poorer classes. This is because the landlord will not pay the charges.

Source G

From the report of an inspection into the living standards of people in Exeter in 1849.

> Heaven helps those who help themselves. The spirit of self-help is the root of all genuine growth in the individual. When help is given to men, it takes away the need of doing it for themselves; and where men are subjected to over-guidance and over-government, the tendency is to make them helpless

Source D

From a book published in 1866.

> A proposal was made for the complete sewerage of the streets. The chief theme of the speakers in opposition to the plan related to saving the pockets of the ratepayers with little regards to the sanitary results.

Source E

From a report on living conditions in Leeds, 1844.

> There is nothing a man so hates as being cleansed against his will, or having his floors swept, his walls whitewashed, his pet dung heaps cleared away. It is a positive fact that many have died from a good washing. All this shows the extreme tenderness with which the work of purification should advance. We prefer to take our chance of cholera than be bullied into health.

Source F

The Times, 1854.

QUESTIONS

2 Read Sources D to G. Match each source with one of the ideas in the list. Explain why they match.

Why were there improvements?

Eventually the government was forced to do something about public health. Edwin Chadwick started the ball rolling.

Step 1 – Edwin Chadwick

Chadwick was a civil servant who was asked to investigate the living conditions and the health of the poor. He became convinced that cleaner towns would lead to less disease and better health. He thought this was a good idea because it would mean ratepayers would have to spend less money on the poor!

We can prevent people becoming ill by building proper sewers and getting rid of cesspools and dung heaps.

The poor are costing us too much - the widows and orphans of men who died through poor health, families whose men cannot work because of sickness – the ratepayers have to pay for all of them. How can I reduce the amount we spend on them?

My report shows that unhealthy living conditions like overcrowding, no sewage disposal and poor diet cause poor health.

We also need a new shape of sewer, not large but small and egg-shaped so it can be constantly flushed by high pressure water. When sewage is left rotting in the sewer it causes bad air which rises and infects people.

If this leads to the poor being healthier they will be able to work harder and the ratepayers will not have to support them.

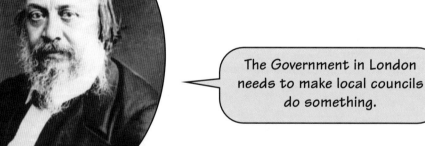

The Government in London needs to make local councils do something.

The rotting sewage and filth everywhere is causing bad air which people are breathing in. All smell is disease.

QUESTIONS

1 List the changes Chadwick wanted to make.

2 What evidence is there that Chadwick believed in the miasma theory?

3 Did Chadwick want to improve conditions because he felt sorry for the poor?

Step 2 – Cholera

At first Chadwick was not able to persuade the government to do anything about public health. You have seen why many people thought that the government had no business to interfere. Cholera changed their minds. Of all the diseases in the 19th century, cholera scared people the most. It could kill thousands of people in a few days and there was no treatment for it. Nearly everyone thought that it was spread by miasma (see Source A). It was a most unpleasant disease – it caused people to lose body fluid and they died of dehydration, 'shrivelled like raisins with blackened extremities, pale, staring, pouring watery fluid from their bowel on the place where they lie'.

Britain had already had one attack of cholera in 1831–2. In 1847 there was news that it was again spreading across Europe and heading towards Britain. This made the government finally act on Chadwick's ideas and pass the 1848 Public Health Act.

The 1848 Public Health Act

- A national General Board of Health was set up.

- In towns where the death rate was very high the General Board of Health could force the local council to set up a local Board of Health to improve water supply and sewerage, and a Medical Officer of Health who had to report dangers to health.

- A local Board of Health and a Medical Officer could also be set up if 10 per cent of the ratepayers petitioned for it.

- Local rates could be levied to pay for the improvements to water supply and sewers.

You can see from the details above that most local councils would not be forced to do anything about water and sewerage. By 1853 Boards of Health were set up in only 103 towns. We have already seen the many reasons why people were against this type of government interference. Most ratepayers were against paying more rates simply to give non-ratepayers benefits they had done nothing to deserve. Many people did not like central government interfering in local affairs.

The national Board of Health was so unpopular that in 1854 it came to an end.

> The chief cause is the poison of atmospheric impurity arising from the accumulation in and around their dwellings of the decomposing remnants of their food and from the impurities given out by their own bodies.
>
> **Source A**

From a report to the government in 1844.

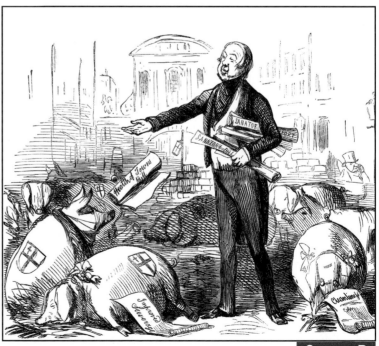

A cartoon published in 1848 about the reaction of ratepayers and local councils to the 1848 Act. It shows the government minister, Lord Morpeth, in the middle, and the Aldermen of local councils who are shown as swine.

Source B

Step 3 – John Snow

By 1854 Britain was again in the middle of a cholera epidemic. This time some progress was made in understanding its causes. John Snow was a famous surgeon who worked in London. (He was the surgeon who used chloroform to help Queen Victoria during childbirth.) His surgery was in Broad Street. In 1854 over 500 people living in Broad Street or nearby streets died from cholera in just ten days. Snow began to investigate. He collected detailed figures about the deaths and the results of his work can be seen in the map and the written source (Sources C and D).

The handle of the Broad Street pump was removed and cholera immediately stopped spreading in the area. It was later discovered that contents from a cesspool, just one metre away, were leaking into the drinking water. Snow had proved that cholera was spread by infected water. This was a remarkable achievement considering Pasteur did not prove his germ theory until 1860 and Koch did not identify the germ that causes cholera until 1883!

Was Snow greeted as a hero? No! Some scientists still believed in the miasma theory. Some even accused Snow of being against sanitary reform because he was claiming that cholera was caused by water rather than by the evil-smelling rubbish that was piled everywhere. They were worried that this took away the argument for cleaning up the rubbish.

> I found that nearly all the deaths had taken place within a short distance of the Broad Street water pump. There were only ten deaths in houses situated nearer to another pump. In five of these cases the deceased persons always used the pump in Broad Street.
>
> There is a brewery in Broad Street. None of the brewer's men died. I called on Mr Huggins, the owner, and he informed me that there were about 70 workmen employed in the brewery. The men are allowed to drink beer, and Mr Huggins is quite certain that they do not drink water at all.
>
> People, of every age and occupation, rich and poor, were being supplied with water containing the sewage of London. Some of this was the excreta from cholera patients who died just before the great outbreak of 1854.

Source C

Extracts from Snow's report 'On the Mode of Communication of Cholera' 1854.

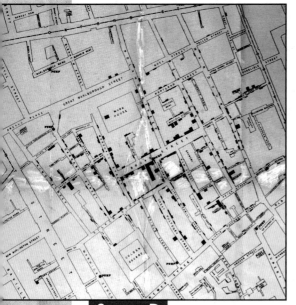

Source D

John Snow's map. The deaths from cholera between 19 August and 30 September 1854 are marked.

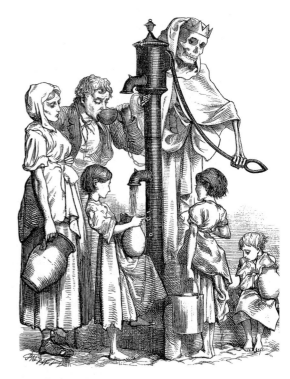

A cartoon published in 1860. It is called 'Death's Dispensary'.

Source E

QUESTIONS

4 Did the artist of the cartoon agree or disagree with Snow? Explain your answer.

5 Imagine you are John Snow. Using Sources C to E write a report explaining (a) how you think cholera is being spread and what evidence you have for your ideas, (b) what you think should be done about it.

Step 4 – The Great Stink of 1858

Snow's discovery did not lead to the government doing something more about public health. Gradually, however, more and more MPs were being persuaded that something should be done. The Great Stink helped in this. The summer of 1858 was hot and dry. The smell coming from the River Thames was unbearable. This affected MPs because the Parliament buildings are right next to the Thames.

What a pity the temperature fell yesterday. Parliament was almost forced to legislate upon the great London nuisance by the force of sheer stench. Some MPs were driven from the library because of the stench which arose from the river.

Source F

From *The Times* newspaper, 18 June 1858.

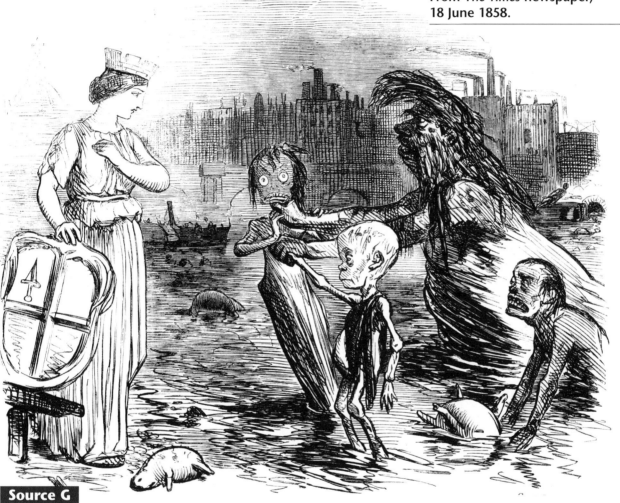

Source G

A cartoon published in July 1858 about the Great Stink.

QUESTIONS

6   What is the message of Source G?

The 1870s – the breakthrough

The big breakthrough came in the 1870s. There were two main reasons why it happened then.

Step 5 – Don't forget Pasteur!

By this time Pasteur's germ theory showing that dirt led to disease was widely accepted and known. It also fitted in with John Snow's work. This made ratepayers more ready to pay to have their towns cleaned up.

Step 6 – Working classes get the vote

The working classes suffered most from poor living conditions. This did not really bother the government because only the rich were able to vote. But in 1867 working-class men living in towns were given the vote. The majority of voters in towns were now working class, so the political parties had to win the support of these workers. One way to do this was to promise better living conditions. In 1874 the Conservatives did this and won the general election because of the votes of the working classes. In 1875 they passed a series of important public health reforms. What is remarkable is that there was hardly any argument about them. This shows how much attitudes had changed since the 1840s. Some historians think that working people getting the vote was the most important reason why governments started to improve public health. They call it 'the death warrant of *laissez-faire*'.

- The Public Health Act made it compulsory for local councils to appoint sanitary inspectors and a medical officer of health, and local councils were given powers to lay sewers and drains, parks and public toilets.

- A Sale of Food and Drugs Act banned adding ingredients that made food a danger to health.

- The Factory Act shortened the hours children and women could be made to work.

- The Artisans' Dwellings Act laid down standards of house building – the size of rooms, sanitation and space between buildings; and gave councils powers to clear slums.

- The River Pollutions Act tried to stop people polluting rivers.

Step 7 – The Great Clean-Up

These laws led to what is known as the Great Clean-Up. This took time but gradually slums were knocked down, clean water was piped to houses, flushing lavatories connected to sewers were built in some houses, cesspools were demolished, yards and streets were paved and dustbins were emptied regularly.

Other factors were also improving the health of the nation.

- Once people had water they could make more use of soap. In 1853 the tax on soap was removed, making it cheaper by one-third. This led to a great increase in the amount of soap being bought and used.

- By the 1890s education was compulsory until the age of 11. This meant that more people could read and could understand the importance of keeping clean.

- The invention of the flushing lavatory meant that human waste was disposed of and not left rotting near to houses.

- The diet of many people improved. More potatoes were eaten. These were cheap and full of vitamin C. The consumption of milk, poultry and eggs increased. This led to healthier people who were less likely to catch diseases.

- Vaccinations to prevent people against diseases were being introduced.

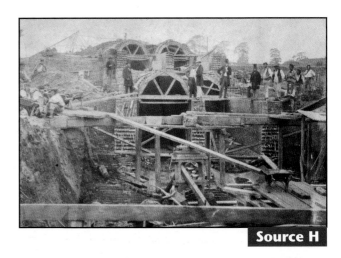

Source H

Sewers being built in the second half of the 19th century.

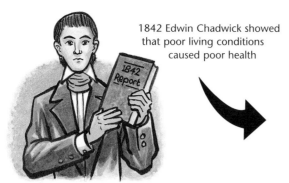

1842 Edwin Chadwick showed that poor living conditions caused poor health

The main reasons for the Great Clean-Up.

Cholera attacks Britain in 1831–32 (31,000 deaths), 1848–49 (62,000 deaths) 1853–54 (31,000 deaths), and 1866 (15,000 deaths)

1854 John Snow shows that disease is spread by infected water.

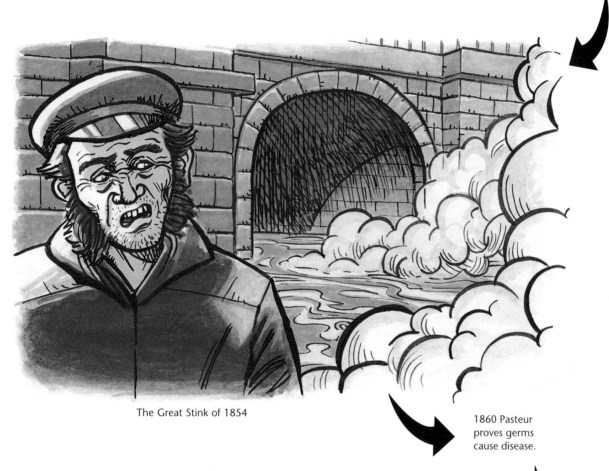

The Great Stink of 1854

1860 Pasteur proves germs cause disease.

1867 The working class get the vote.

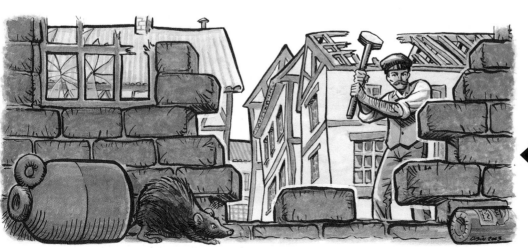

The Great Clean-Up of 1870s. Pulling down of slums, provision of clean water and proper sewers and drains now begins

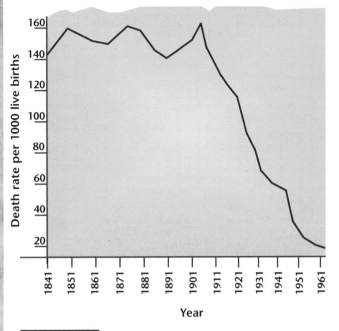

The infant death rate in England and Wales between 1841 and 1961.

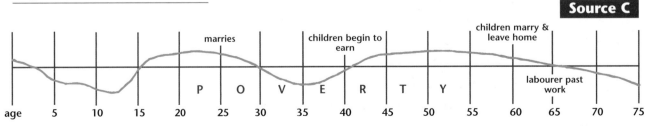

Liberal Reforms

The improvements made in the 19th century must not be exaggerated. While water supplies, sewers and drains were improved, progress was slow. It also became clear that clean water and good sewers and drains were not enough. Many people were still very poor. They lived in terrible conditions and died from diseases like tuberculosis. Source A shows that the infant death rate had hardly changed during the second half of the 19th century. The problem that now had to be tackled was poverty. People who were poor could not afford decent housing, enough food or medical help. There were certain groups who were particularly in need of help – young children, the unemployed, those who were sick and could not work, mothers whose husbands had died, the old who no longer had jobs.

Why the government acted

- In 1900 it was found that 40 per cent of the men volunteering to fight in the Boer War were too unhealthy and unfit to be soldiers. This was caused by poor diet, living in overcrowded housing and smoke pollution.

- Charles Booth investigated the poor of London. He found that 30 per cent of Londoners did not have enough money to buy the basics – food, shelter and clothing. He also discovered that 85 per cent of those living in poverty were poor because they were unemployed or their wages were so low. This meant that their poverty was not their fault. Booth published a series of reports between 1889 and 1903, which made his findings well known.

- Seebohm Rowntree found a similar situation in York. Nearly 30 per cent of the population had barely enough money for the basics like food, rent, fuel and clothing. He produced what he called a poverty line, which showed when in their lives people were most likely to be poor.

Source B

A photograph of the inside of a working class home in the 1890s. Many families lived in single rooms like this one.

Rowntree's poverty line. If you were below the line you did not have enough money for food, shelter and clothing. If you were above the line you had just enough to survive.

How people were helped

Mothers and babies

1902 Training for midwives was made compulsory

1907 The local Medical Officer of Health had to be told when a baby was born. A Health Visitor then visited the mother to teach her how to protect her baby's health

Growing children

1906 Local councils were given the power to provide free school meals for children. By 1914, over 158,000 children were receiving a free meal

1907 School children were regularly inspected by nurses or doctors

1912 School clinics were set up to give children free medical treatment

The old

1908 Everyone over the age of 70 was paid an old-age pension

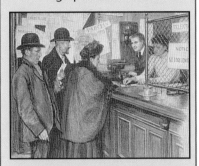

A photo of people collecting the first old-age pensions.

The sick and the unemployed

1909 Labour exchanges were set up to help people find work

1911 A compulsory insurance scheme was set up for all low-paid workers. They, their employers, and the government paid money into the scheme. When the workers fell ill and could not work they were given money every week. They were also given free medical care when they were sick

1912 The above scheme was extended to help unemployed workers in some industries like shipbuilding where unemployment was seasonal

The homeless and people living in slums

1909 Back-to-back houses were forbidden. Builders had to follow proper standards when building houses

1919 The government helped local councils to provide 'Homes fit for heroes' for the soldiers returning from the First World War

QUESTIONS

1 These reforms are very different from the public health reforms of the 19th century. Which of the following apply to the 19th-century reforms, and which apply to the reforms of the Liberal government?

(a) The government had a duty to help the poor.

(b) People knew that germs caused disease.

(c) Groups like the young, the old and the unemployed needed most help.

(d) The main problem was dirt and polluted water.

(e) Poverty led to poor health.

(f) Many poor people could not help being poor.

(g) The important thing was to make people stronger and healthier.

The National Health Service

Despite the reforms at the beginning of the 20th century there was still much to do. In the 1940s, after the Second World War, a Labour Government established the Welfare State. This involved the government providing services and support to make sure that everyone had a reasonable standard of living. An important part of these reforms was the setting up of the National Health Service.

Why was the National Health Service established?

Most people could not afford proper medical care

About half the population were covered by health insurance. Doctors and hospitals charged patients fees and most people not covered by insurance could not afford them. This meant that they did not receive proper medical care and did not benefit from the many medical advances of the time. Many depended on treatments such as: 'My husband's father used to burn camphor on a hot shovel and blow it about the room when his children were coughing.'

The insurance system was failing

In the 1930s Britain suffered from high unemployment. Many of those who lost their jobs could no longer pay their insurance contributions. By 1934, four million people were behind with their payments. The system set up by the Liberals was falling apart.

Death rate of infants rising

There was evidence that in towns such as Wigan, where unemployment was high, the death rate of infants was rising. It was clear that the poor needed more help.

The Second World War

This changed peoples' attitudes in many ways:

- Evacuation
  During the war many working-class children from inner city areas were evacuated to the countryside. Middle-class families who took them in were shocked when they saw how unhealthy, under-nourished, dirty and poorly clothed they were. This persuaded many people that something had to be done after the war had ended.

- People wanted to build a better society
  During the war people had made many sacrifices. There was a general hope that a better society could be built after the war. One aspect of this would be good health care for everyone.

- Working together
  During the war people had worked together. Differences of social class had often been ignored. This created a feeling that everyone, not just the rich, should have good health care.

- During the war the government had provided free medical treatment to keep people well for the war effort. People had become used to getting free medical services.

The Beveridge Report, 1942

During the war Sir William Beveridge was asked to produce a report recommending what should be done after the war was over. In 1942 he produced his report. He said that war should be declared on:

- WANT (poverty). This would be fought by everyone in work paying a weekly contribution. In return they would get benefits when they were sick, unemployed, old and pregnant.

- DISEASE. This was to be fought by setting up a National Health Service (NHS). It would be paid for out of taxes and be free to everyone. Hospitals were nationalised and the NHS provided general practitioners (GPs), hospitals, doctors and nurses, midwives and dentists.

In the 1945 election the Labour Party promised to carry out Beveridge's ideas. This was one of the main reasons people voted the Labour Party into power.

Opposition to the setting up of the NHS

There was some opposition to the idea of the NHS. This came from:

- Doctors who were worried that if they were employed by the NHS they would lose their freedom.

- Doctors who wanted to carry on treating private patients who paid them fees.

- Local councils which ran the hospitals. They lost control of the hospitals.

- People who still believed that others were poor because they were lazy or spent their money on drink. They asked why should such people be helped?

- Those who believed that if people were helped by the state in this way they would come to depend on it completely and would be unable to look after themselves and their families. People would get used to getting something for nothing, and this was not good for them – it could make them lazy.

The doctors were won over when they were allowed to keep their private patients. Soon, they supported the NHS as much as everyone else.

In 1948 the NHS was founded. The most immediate result was that millions of people got free dentures, glasses and hearing aids. Over eight million people who had never seen a doctor now received proper care. A big hospital building programme was started. Nurses and doctors in hospitals were amazed by the amount of new medical supplies they had. For decades the NHS was an outstanding success.

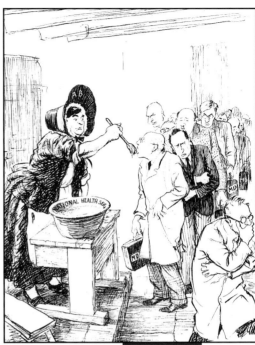

Source A

A cartoon published in 1948. The woman represents Aneurin Bevan, the government minister who introduced the NHS. He is giving the doctors their medicine. They complain 'It all tastes awful'.

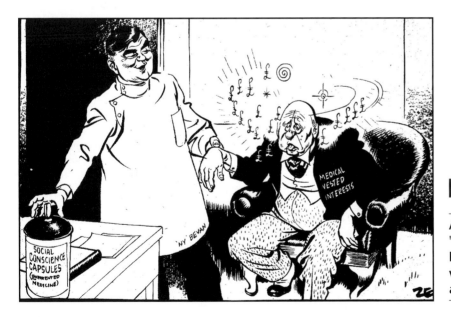

Source B

A cartoon published in 1945. 'Vested interests' means those had by people who are doing well from things as they are and do not want change.

QUESTIONS

1 Study Sources A and B. Are they supporting or attacking the NHS? Explain your answer.

Surgery in the early 19th century

On pages 142–3 are three written descriptions and one illustration of surgery in the 19th century. Study them carefully and then answer the questions at the bottom of page 143.

For the exam you will need to know:

☑ The problems faced by surgeons and their patients

☑ How anaesthetics were developed by James Simpson and others

☑ How antiseptics were developed by Joseph Lister

☑ How the problem of bleeding was overcome

☑ Why Florence Nightingale is important.

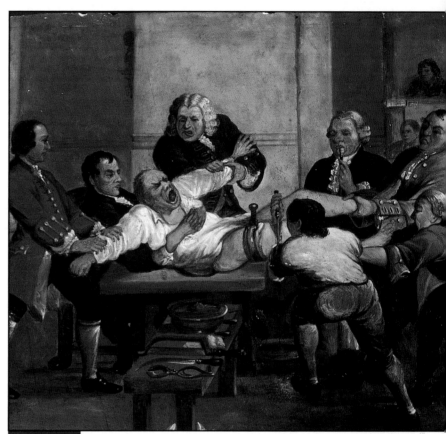

Source A

A painting of surgery around 1800.

I remember very well the horrors of surgery. The most difficult moment was that of the first incision. But there were always close at hand the house-surgeons ready to grasp the patient if necessary in such a way that he could not easily interrupt the work of the surgeon ... Operations were done as rapidly as possible. I think I have seen large amputations done in less than a minute.

I remember an operation upon a young man for the removal of a large cancerous growth on the end of his tongue. The operation was done by a short, quick stroke of the knife which removed the outer half of the tongue. Of course, the bleeding was quite free. Dr Warren stepped back to the furnace, where the hot iron was. At a look from Dr Warren the house-surgeon quickly slipped both of his hands over the patient's eyes and the cautery was instantly applied to the whole bleeding surface. The patient suddenly jerked backwards.

A description of surgery in the 1840s by Dr Samuel Abbot.

Source B

Often one came upon an empty ward with a little notice pasted upon the glass door: 'Ward closed for cleaning'. We knew what that meant, blood poisoning had broken out. We students were allowed to go from the dissecting and post-mortem room to attend midwifery cases. True there was a faded notice-board on which was written 'Gentlemen who are dissecting should wash their hands in chlorinated soda solution before going to their cases.' But I never knew of anyone doing it, nor did we have the least idea of the reason for the notice.

I remember the house surgeon with his threaded needles dangling from his coat, the silken threads sweeping the well-worn cloth. I see the coat now, faded with age, stained with blood and spotted with pus.

The 'ward sponge' was simply wrung out in warm water and passed from case to case. It was the fashion then to clean up ulcers, and nothing did the work so well as the sponge.

Source C

A description of operations in the 1870s by a medical student.

I brought down the edge of the knife and cut with a sawing motion. My assistant pressed on the numerous cut arteries with his hand. I now cut down close along the bone, and then made a single cut upon the head of the bone, which with a loud noise popped from its socket. Is seemed at first as if the bleeding vessels which supplied so many jets of blood could never all be closed. But in the course of a few minutes the bleeding was restrained by the application of ten or twelve ligatures.

Source D

Description by Dr Syme of the amputation of a leg in 1830s.

QUESTIONS

1   Make a list of all the problems facing the surgeon and the patient during these operations.

2   For each problem explain what, if anything, was done about it.

You have probably managed to identify three problems: pain, infection and bleeding.

Pain

Although opium and alcohol were used to make the patient drowsy or to dull the pain they were not very effective. In any case, it was not very easy operating on a patient who was drunk. Surgeons in Scotland used the Moore's clamp (see Source E). For most people surgery was unrelieved agony and many died from the shock of the pain. This all made speed important – it was obviously better to be in agony for one minute than for ten minutes. As far as most people were concerned, the quickest surgeon was the best surgeon. Some could amputate a leg in under a minute! One of the most famous was Robert Liston. When he was ready to operate he would shout to students who had gathered to watch 'Time me, gentlemen, time me!'

Surgeons were the stars of their day. Operating day was a weekly show with students and the public flocking in to watch. During operations Liston held his bloody knife between his teeth so as to free both hands. In one case he amputated the leg of a patient in two minutes, but in his hurry he cut off the patient's testicles as well. On another occasion he amputated a leg so quickly that he also cut off his assistant's thumb, who died later from the infection. He also slashed through the coat tails of a spectator, who was so terrified that the knife had pierced his genitals that he dropped dead from fright.

Infection

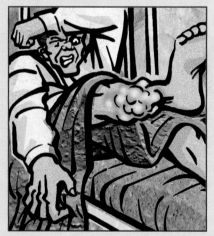

Many patients survived the operation but died later from infection. Once the body had been opened up it was very easy for the wound or the blood to become infected. Remember, Pasteur had not yet discovered that germs cause disease and so very few hygiene precautions were taken. Gangrene and blood poisoning were common – they could have both been easily treated by antibiotics such as penicillin but, of course, surgeons did not know this. The usual pattern was that a day or two after the operation the wound would become red and inflamed. It would then become septic and fill with pus. The infection then spread to the rest of the body and eventually the patient would die. Some doctors thought infection was caused by bad air and recommended operations be done in a current of wind!

In most hospitals the death rate following amputation was between 25 and 50 per cent. Of the 2089 amputations performed outside hospital only 10 per cent died. James Simpson, who did a survey of amputations, concluded 'A man laid on the operating table in hospital is exposed to more chances of death than was the English soldier on the battlefield of Waterloo.'

Bleeding

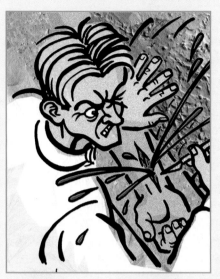

When patients were operated on they bled. If nothing was done about this they would bleed to death. It was common to tie blood vessels with ligatures (remember Paré doing this?) made of thread or catgut. However, sometimes the ligature cut through the blood vessel, or the catgut would slip, and on other occasions the ligature was dirty and caused infection. In any case, ligatures only helped after operations had finished. To carry out long operations surgeons needed a way of coping with bleeding during the operation.

Attempts were made as early as the 17th century to transfuse blood from animals into humans. It didn't work because the human body will reject animal blood. In the early 19th century transfusions were carried out from human to human but they worked only if the people had the same blood groups (different blood groups were not known about then). The blood often clotted and the patient died; often the blood was infected giving the same result.

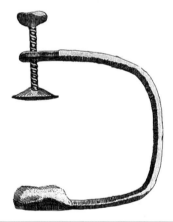

Source A

Moore's clamp. Pain is caused by the nerves sending messages to the brain. The screw was twisted into the limb squeezing the nerves to stop the messages from the nerves to the brain. However, as the screw was tightened it caused as much pain as the operation.

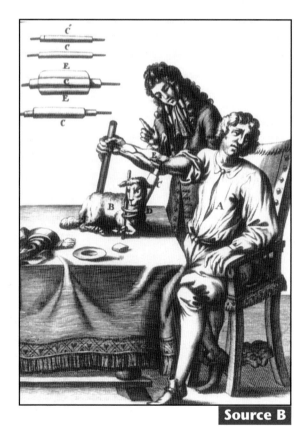

Source B

A seventeenth-century drawing of blood transfusion from a lamb to a human.

If these three problems were not solved, operations would not go beyond fractures and amputations – just as in Paré's time. The range of operations attempted was narrow. The most common was amputation, but some surgeons did try more ambitious operations. In 1809 a woman had a huge ovarian cyst removed. It took 25 minutes to remove the 15 pound water-filled tumour. The patient sang hymns to drown the pain. But most operations were simple amputations. Pain, infection and bleeding all limited what surgeons could do.

Surgery makes progress

Fighting pain

The first problem to be tackled was that of pain.

The road to chloroform

In 1795 Humphrey Davy, a scientist, discovered that laughing gas relieved the pain from an inflamed gum. He wrote that it 'seemed capable of destroying pain' and 'may be used with advantage during surgical operations'. But nobody followed up his ideas.

In 1844 Horace Wells, an American dentist, went to a fair where laughing gas was being demonstrated. He wondered whether it would make having a tooth out painless. So he tried it. As he recovered consciousness he exclaimed 'A new era of tooth-pulling'. He built some bellows that blew the gas into the patient's mouth through a tube. When he tried a demonstration in front of medical students it went badly wrong and the patient was in agony. He was discredited and later committed suicide.

In 1846 John Warren, an American doctor, carried out the first operation under anaesthetic using ether. A small tumour from the patient's neck was removed while the patient was unconscious.

In 1846 Robert Liston used ether when amputating a diseased leg. When the patient regained consciousness he didn't realise the operation had been done and he asked 'When are you going to begin?' Liston's operation became famous and other surgeons began to use ether.

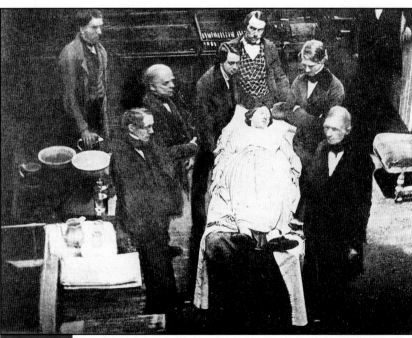

A daguerreotype of John Warren carrying out the first operation under anaesthetic.

Source A

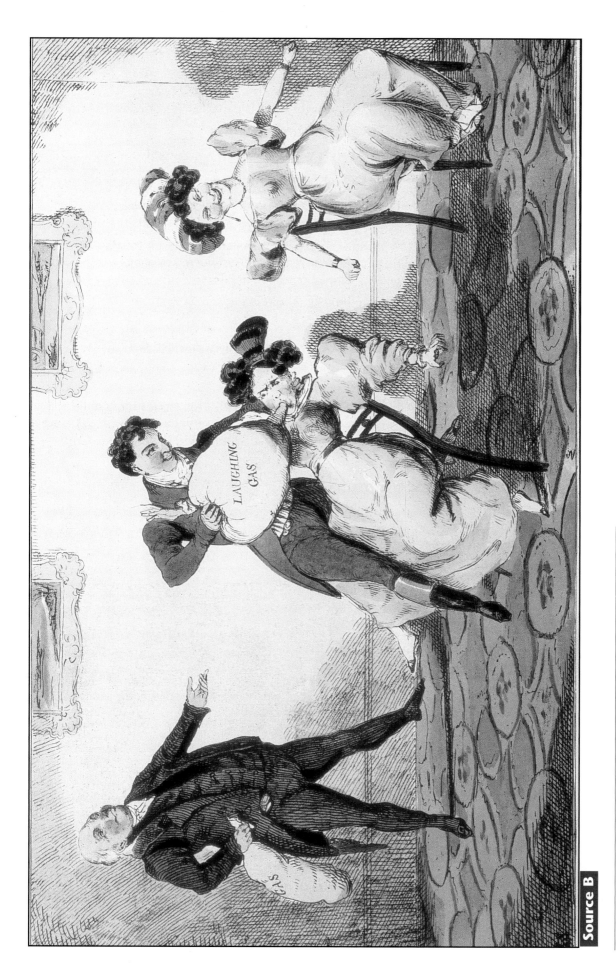

This cartoon from 1830 shows that laughing gas was not taken seriously as an anaesthetic.

James Simpson and chloroform

James Simpson was born in 1811 in Scotland and trained as a doctor at Edinburgh University. In 1839 he became Professor of Midwifery at Edinburgh. He was particularly concerned about the suffering of women during childbirth.

Problems with ether

Simpson used ether for childbirth but there were problems with it:

- It was transported in a large, heavy glass bottle – very difficult for a doctor to carry around with him.
- It had an unpleasant small that lingered over the patients for a long time.
- It irritated the lungs and made people sick.
- It irritated the eyes.
- If it was held close to a flame it could catch fire.

Source A describes how Simpson experimented in 1847 to find an alternative to ether.

Within days Simpson had used chloroform during childbirth and for an operation on a boy with an infected elbow. He poured the chloroform on a handkerchief and held it over the patient's face.

Opposition!

You might think that everyone would welcome anaesthetics like chloroform. However, there were some people who opposed its use.

Having inhaled several substances but without much effect, it occurred to Dr Simpson to try chloroform which he had rejected because of its great weight. The small bottle of chloroform was searched for and recovered from beneath a heap of waste paper. And with each glass newly filled, the inhalers continued. Immediately they became bright-eyed and very happy. And then crash! On awakening Dr Simpson's first thought was 'This is far stronger and better than ether.'

Source A

Professor Miller, a neighbour of Simpson's, who called on Simpson the morning after the experiment, in 1847.

A portable chloroform inhaler developed by John Snow in the 1850s.

Some people thought it was cowardly to have an anaesthetic. One senior army officer said it was much better 'to hear a man bawl lustily than to see him sink silently into the grave'.

Some doctors argued that it was not necessary to use a general anaesthetic for child birth and minor operations.

Some people opposed it for religious reasons. They pointed out that the Bible said that childbirth was meant to be painful. If God had wanted it to be painless, he would have made it so. Surgeons were going against God's will.

Some doctors were worried that patients would be given too much chloroform and would die. They said more tests were needed so the correct dosage could be agreed.
In 1848 a 15-year-old girl died from an overdose of chloroform while having a toenail removed.

The death rate from operations went up when anaesthetics were first used! They encouraged doctors to carry out longer and more complicated operations and patients died from infection and bleeding.

Some people claimed that chloroform was untested – it might have nasty side effects that had not yet been discovered.

Source B

Acceptance

In April 1853 anaesthetics took a big step forward when Queen Victoria used chloroform for the birth of her eighth child. She wrote in her journal 'The effect was soothing, quieting and delightful beyond measure.' If it was all right for the Queen, then it was all right for everyone else!

Anaesthetics get better ...

Since Simpson's time anaesthetics have developed in many ways

- Deep unconsciousness always carries risks. A local anaesthetic that just dulled the pain in the area being operated, without making the patient unconscious, was needed. Scientists managed to extract cocaine from coca leaves and, in the 1880s, it was used for the first time. Today synthetic substances such as xylocaine are used.

- Surgeons didn't just need a patient to be asleep. They also required the muscles in the body to be relaxed. This required a lot of anaesthetic which could be dangerous and could take days to wear off. What was needed was a muscle-relaxing drug that could be given alongside the anaesthetic. The South American arrow-poison curare was the answer. The only problem was that it relaxed the muscles that controlled breathing, causing patients to stop breathing. In the 1930s artificial respiration was developed and curare could be used.

- From 1902 anaesthetics were injected through the skin and into the blood vessels.

...but cause problems

- Chloroform led to surgeons conducting deeper and longer operations. This increased the chances of the patient being infected and the death rate in operations went up!

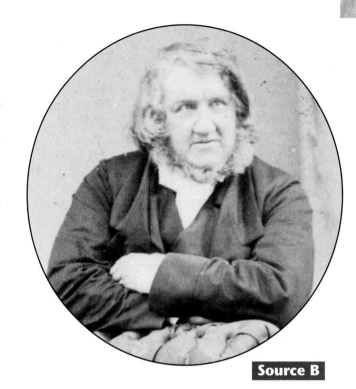

Source B

James Simpson

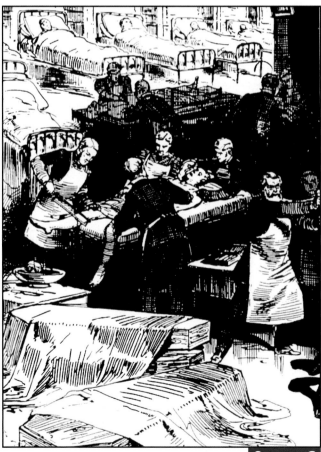

A cartoon from the 1870s when anaesthetics were coming into general use. Does the cartoon support or oppose the use of anaesthetics?

Source C

Joseph Lister and antiseptics

Lister was born in 1827 in Yorkshire. He became an assistant surgeon in Edinburgh in 1854 and Professor of Surgery at Glasgow University in 1860. He found infection rife in the operating theatre at Glasgow. Many patients developed gangrene, which most doctors blamed on miasma or bad air. Lister was appalled by the filthy state of the wards because by this time he suspected that there was a connection between dirt and disease. He insisted on the wards being kept much cleaner but there was not much improvement in the death rate.

In 1865 Lister read some of Pasteur's early writings. These told him that gangrene or rotting was caused by airborne bacteria. Remember this was at a time before Pasteur had fully formed his germ theory of disease. However, Lister made the mental leap – it was not the air that caused the infection of his patients, it was the microbes in it. Somehow they had to be killed before they reached the wounds of the patients. It did not take Lister long to come up with an answer. As Source B shows, he had already been thinking along these lines and he had a solution to hand.

Lister tried out his theory on patients with compound fractures. These are fractures where the bone has pierced the skin, leaving a wound in need of dressing. These wounds often became infected. He smeared the carbolic acid onto the wound and then covered it with a cloth soaked in carbolic. This was covered with tin foil to stop the liquid evaporating. When he removed the dressing a scab had formed with no sign of infection. In all, he used this method on 11 patients – nine of them survived, an unheard of survival rate at that time.

Years	Total cases	Lived	Died	Mortality %
1864-66 (without antiseptics)	35	19	16	45.7
1867-70 (with antiseptics)	40	34	6	15.0

Source C

Lister's results using carbolic acid.

Lister knew he had to publicise his new ideas. By 1867 he had written a paper and given a talk to the British Medical Association about his antiseptic methods. He also kept improving his methods.

- He developed antiseptic ligatures for tying up wounds

- He also developed a carbolic spray which was used in operating theatres to try to kill the germs in the air

- He also realised that germs could be carried into wounds by the fingers and instruments of the doctor, so he insisted that surgeons wash their hands and instruments with carbolic before operations.

Antiseptics had long been discussed and were widely used. Greek medicine had used wine and vinegar in wound care, sanitarians like Florence Nightingale insisted on spotless conditions in hospitals. But such disinfective moves were not based on an understanding of bacteria. They were merely attempts to fight contagious diseases. Lister did not invent antiseptic surgery, he made it effective, he made it routine, he made it famous, and thus made surgery safe.

Source A

A recent historian.

In the course of the year 1864 I was much struck with an account of the remarkable effects produced by carbolic acid upon the sewage of the town of Carlisle. It prevented all odour from the lands covered with the sewage and also destroyed the parasites which usually infest cattle fed upon such pastures. The idea of using carbolic acid for the treatment of compound fractures naturally occurred to me.

Source B

Lister writing in 1867.

Opposition!

Like Simpson, Lister's methods were opposed.

- Some doctors denied that there were germs in the air that caused disease – it was only in 1867 that Pasteur carried out his experiments proving the existence of airborne germs and it took him some time to convince everyone that he was right. One professor mocked Lister, saying 'Where are these little beasts? Show them to us, and we shall believe in them. Has anyone seen them yet?'

- Lister kept changing his methods. This was to make improvements – for example he knew doctors and nurses did not like working with carbolic acid so he tried to find another substance, less unpleasant. But to other doctors it looked as if he changed his methods because they were not working.

- Many doctors believed that speed was the most important factor in surgery. The use of carbolic acid slowed them down and was therefore seen as a nuisance – even dangerous.

- Surgeons who copied Lister's methods were often not as careful as Lister. Their results were not as good and so they thought his methods did not work.

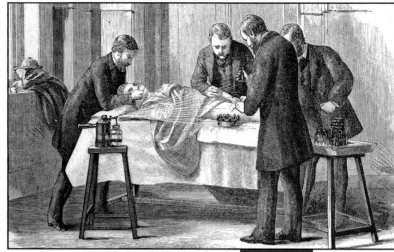

Source D

A drawing of Lister's carbolic spray being used in an operation. The doctor standing by the patient's head is holding a handkerchief soaked in chloroform over the patient's head.

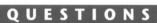

QUESTIONS

1 Go back to Source A. Do you agree with the last sentence of this source? It makes several points about Lister. Make sure you comment on them all.

Lister's methods

As news of the survival rate of Lister's patients, and of Pasteur's and Koch's discoveries, spread other surgeons accepted his methods. Lister's methods were copied in hospitals all over Europe and in America, but they were not perfect. His methods were a mixture of the old and the new.

- He only rinsed his hands in carbolic, he did not scrub them. Germs were left in the lines of the skin. An experiment in 1897 showed that carbolic acid was not killing the germs on surgeons' hands. It was abandoned. Koch had shown that chemicals were less effective than heat for sterilising instruments and boiling became the usual method of sterilisation. In 1890 Lister abandoned the carbolic spray.

- Lister continued to operate in his ordinary clothes. Others developed face masks, rubber gloves and surgical gowns.

- Lister did not develop any new operations. Nearly all his operations were on broken bones and surface tumours. However, within a few years of Lister's death, surgeons were opening up the body and operating on internal organs such as the liver and the pancreas. Lister helped make all this possible.

> Everything was soaked in carbolic, hands, instruments and patients' skins. Huge quarts of the precious fluid were everywhere around. The whole scene of an operation was covered in its spray, which dispersed its globules into every nook and cranny of the wound. Our faces and coat-sleeves often dripped with it.
>
> It was a relief to us all when the spray was abandoned. It was costly and cumbersome and often broke down. Carbolic acid made sad work with our hands which were always rough and cracked.

Source E

From the memoirs of a doctor who worked with Lister.

THE 18TH TO 20TH CENTURIES

The nurses too conspired against him. They thought the be-all of their mission was for the patients to have shining faces, tidy lockers and to say their prayers often. They resented the extra work antiseptics gave them, the endless washings of basins.

One of the surgeons could always raise a laugh by telling anyone who came into the operating room to shut the door quickly lest one of Mr Lister's microbes should come in.

Source F

From a doctor who worked with Lister.

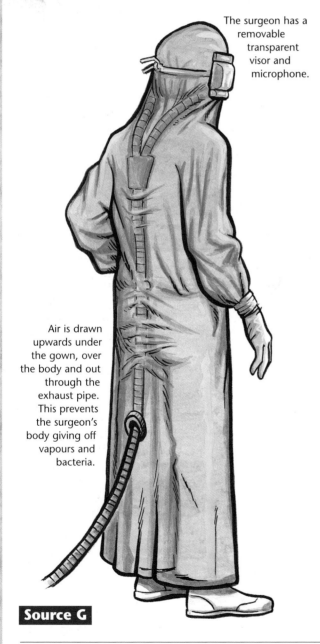

The surgeon has a removable transparent visor and microphone.

Air is drawn upwards under the gown, over the body and out through the exhaust pipe. This prevents the surgeon's body giving off vapours and bacteria.

Source G

A surgeon using the Charnley–Howarth Body Exhaust System.

Aseptic surgery

Lister had made antiseptic surgery (taking precautions against germs) widespread. It was a small move from there to aseptic surgery (the complete elimination of bacteria where an operation is taking place).

Remember that Lister conducted his operations in his everyday clothes. Gradually, special clothing was developed for surgeons.

- Rubber gloves started to be used in the 1840s but were opposed at first by supporters of Lister because they claimed that as the antiseptics took care of the germs in the wound, gloves were not needed. They were made popular in the 1880s by the American surgeon William Halsted. His theatre sister was suffering from eczema on her hands caused by carbolic acid. He urged her to wear rubber gloves and they worked perfectly. The gloves were sterilised with steam, as were all bandages and threads.

- In 1897 a facemask was worn for the first time during an operation. Source G shows the methods used in the 1970s to keep surgeons germ free.

QUESTIONS

1 Carbolic acid was very unpopular. What reasons for opposition to Lister's methods can you find in Sources E and F that are not mentioned above?

2 Did people oppose Simpson and Lister for the same reasons?

The problem of bleeding

Blood groups

Bleeding during operations was last of the three problems to be tackled. Although blood transfusions did take place in the 19th century (as Source A shows) most were unsuccessful. The turning point came with the discovery of blood groups. In 1901 Karl Landsteiner discovered that humans had three types of blood which he called A, B and 0. In the following year group AD was discovered, and other groups have been found since. Only some of these could be transferred from a patient of one group to another.

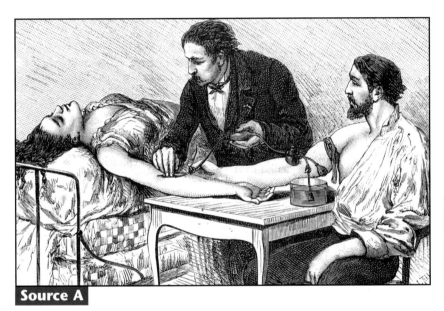

Source A

A successful blood transfusion given to a woman after childbirth in 1882.

Storing blood

It took some time for blood transfusions to be widely used because they had to be from person to person – both the patient and the donor had to be present. When doctors tried to store blood it clotted. During the First World War many soldiers suffered the most dreadful wounds. Many bled to death because it was not possible to have donors on the spot.

- In 1914 it was found that sodium citrate stopped drawn blood clotting in a syringe. This gave doctors a little more flexibility.

- The real breakthrough was when blood cells were separated from the liquid part and stored in a glucose solution. Bottles of corpuscles could be stored in bottles and diluted with a saline solution when needed.

- Large blood banks were developed in the US and Britain during the Second World War and today Britain has a National Blood Transfusion Service that stores and distributes blood across the country.

War and surgery

Plastic surgery had been attempted for hundreds of years. Ancient texts from India show that they reconstructed noses and we have seen the advances made by Paré. However, the problem of pain meant that surgeons had to work at speed and with little accuracy. There was also the problem of infection. Real advances began during the First World War. Never before had soldiers been subjected to such heavy shelling and surgeons were faced with increasing numbers of horrible facial injuries. The rifles used caused big entry wounds. A soldier shot side-on would lose his nose and face, and perhaps be blinded.

> I saw one soldier with his jaw clean blown away. Others were vomiting great gobs of blood, men without noses, and their brains throbbing through open scalps, men without faces.

Source B

From a diary of a nurse who worked on the Western Front in 1915.

> Hideous is the only word for these smashed faces; the socket with some twisted slit, with an eyelash or two hanging on feebly, the skewed mouth which results from the loss of a jaw, far the worst is when the nose is missing altogether.
>
> Without surgery his face would be worse than it is, and yet in his mirror he is faced with a gargoyle. Suppose he is married. Could any woman come near that gargoyle without repugnance? His children? Why, a child would run screaming from such a sight.

Source C

An orderly working at a hospital during the First World War.

Skilled skin-grafting has reconstructed a something which has two small holes that are his nostrils, but the something is not a nose.

Sometimes full reconstructions of faces are not possible and masks, known as Tin Faces, are constructed to cover large facial defects.

My broken and septic teeth were extracted and my wound cleaned. The problem then was how to reunite the broken fragments of my lower jaw which were still hanging loosely in my mouth. The solution was to set the broken bones of the lower jaw and then cement it to the upper jaw which acted as a splint. As most of my lower jaw had gone, I was shown an album of photographs of handsome young men and asked to choose the chin I would like to have.

Source D

Because of the danger of infection surgeons were moved out to hospitals near the front so that they could operate quickly. A new hospital with over a thousand beds was set up in Sidcup in England to specialise in facial injuries. Over 11,000 operations were carried out.

QUESTIONS

1 **Look at the three accounts from the First World War in Source D, then make lists of what the surgeons were able to do for the soldiers, and what they were not able to do.**

Hector McIndoe worked at the Sidcup hospital in the First World War. During the Second World War he set up his own unit in East Grinstead and developed plastic surgery further. He treated over 4,000 patients. Many were aircrew with horrific facial burns. He did much to reconstruct the damaged faces and hands.

The face was like a mask. At a distance he looked the same; the marks of McIndoe's work were visible. The skin on his face was entirely new, taken from the flaps cut from his arms and legs; where the patches fitted over the bone structure it was shiny and pink, and the seams of each different patch were plainly visible.

Source E

Description of a fighter pilot who was badly burned in the Battle of Britain. This account is based on the memories of his parents and friends.

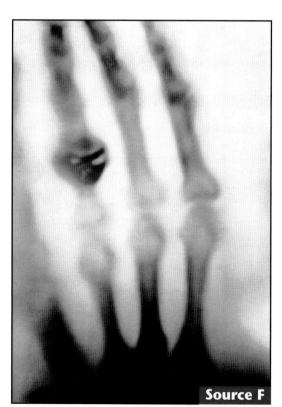

Source F

X-rays

In 1895 Karl Wilhelm Rontgen was experimenting with rays when he found some that passed through his cardboard cover. He beamed the ray on his wife's hand and found he could see her bones and rings highlighted against the surrounding flesh. His discovery made newspaper headlines. There were fears of Peeping Toms with 'X-ray eyes' peering through women's underclothes, and one firm advertised X-ray-proof knickers!

Soon X-rays were being used to scan for gallstones, fractures and, during wartime, bullets in the body. By the 1920s mass chest X-ray screening was developed and X-rays had become a valuable method of diagnosis.

One of the first X-ray photographs taken by Rontgen

Modern surgery

Surgery at the end of the 20th century had come along way since the time of Lister and Simpson.

Surgeons can now work calmly inside the heart while it is disconnected. This means that the patient's blood circulation has to be maintained with a machine to keep supplying oxygen to the rest of the body.

The real heart is stopped with an electric shock. It is cooled down and the body temperature lowered to 28 degrees so that it needs less oxygen. At the end of the operation the heart is started with electrical help.

Transplanting of organs is now common. The problem of the body rejecting transplanted organs was overcome by drugs in the 1960s. In 1967 in South Africa, Dr Christian Barnard completed the first heart transplant when he sewed a heart from a 24-year-old woman who had died in a car accident into a 54-year-old woman. She died just 18 days later, but by the 1980s hundreds of heart transplants were being carried out each year with two-thirds of the patients living for five years or more.

Now, livers, kidneys, the pancreas and marrow-bone (to cure blood diseases like leukaemia) can all be transplanted.

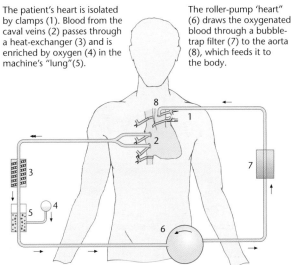

The patient's heart is isolated by clamps (1). Blood from the caval veins (2) passes through a heat-exchanger (3) and is enriched by oxygen (4) in the machine's "lung"(5).

The roller-pump 'heart' (6) draws the oxygenated blood through a bubble-trap filter (7) to the aorta (8), which feeds it to the body.

Source G

How a heart-lung machine works.

It is terrifying to think what will happen when the mystery of organ transference has been solved. Anybody would be able to go into his local organ bank and trade in a weak heart or a feeble brain for a better one, or a cirrhotic liver for a healthier one.

Source H

A look into the possible future.

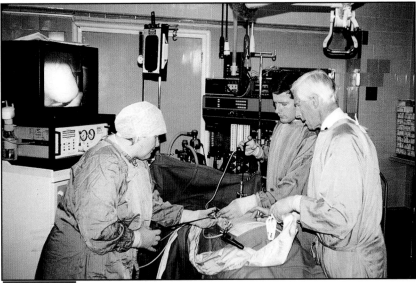

Source I

Keyhole surgery involves operations being carried out through small telescopes inserted into the body through tiny incisions. The surgeons are guided by images from the telescopes of the inside of the body which are shown on the monitors.

EXAM PRACTICE QUESTIONS

(a) Describe the problems that faced surgeons in the early nineteenth century.

(b) Explain why some people opposed the use of antiseptics and anaesthetics.

(c) How far had problems in surgery been overcome by the end of the nineteenth century?

CASE STUDY

Who was the more important – Florence Nightingale or Mary Seacole?

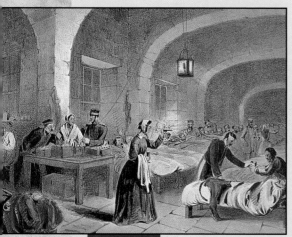

A painting from 1855 of Florence Nightingale in Scutari Hospital. She was popularly known as 'the lady with the lamp' because it was claimed she walked the wards at night making sure the wounded soldiers were comfortable.

You have already seen how bad many hospitals were in the 19th century. They were places to stay clear of, hotbeds of infection. If you went into one you were more likely to catch an infection than be successfully treated. The rich did not go near them – they had their operations done at home. One historian has called them 'gateways to death'. Lister made an important contribution towards making hospitals cleaner and safer places but much work was also done by nurses such as Florence Nightingale and Mary Seacole.

The legend of Florence Nightingale

You are now going to investigate how true the impression given by Sources A and B was. You are also going to tackle two other questions.

■ Was being 'the Lady of the Lamp' Florence Nightingale's most important contribution to medicine?

■ Was she really more important than Mary Seacole?

Q1 What impression of Florence Nightingale do Sources A and B give?

A painting from 1856. It is called 'The Mission of Mercy: Florence Nightingale Receiving the Wounded at Scutari'.

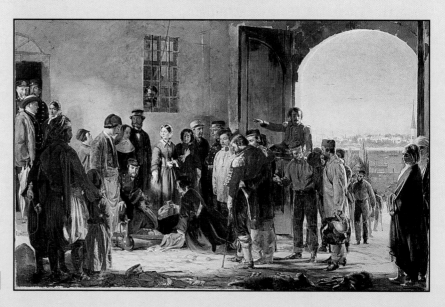

Florence Nightingale's story

Nightingale was born into a wealthy family in 1820. When she announced that God wanted her to become a nurse and care for the sick, her parents were horrified. At that time nursing was not a respectable job. Nurses were poorly paid, had little training, and were often general 'dogsbodies'. Source C gives you a good idea of the attitudes of the time towards nurses. When she was 31 she was allowed to be trained as a nurse in Germany. She worked in several hospitals before becoming superintendent of nurses at King's College Hospital in London.

In 1854 the course of Nightingale's life changed completely. In that year the Crimean War broke out between Britain and Russia. William Russell, the reporter for *The Times* newspaper, sent back reports from the front describing the terrible conditions suffered by the soldiers, especially those who were wounded. Russell's reports led to a public outcry for something to be done. Sidney Herbert, the member of the government responsible for the army, was a good friend of Nightingale. They agreed that she would take a group of 38 nurses to Scutari.

Florence Nightingale at Scutari

Nightingale arrived at Scutari on 4 November 1854. She was appalled by what she saw at Scutari Hospital. Within six months she reduced the death rate in the hospital from 40 per cent to 2 per cent. When she returned to Britain in 1856 she was a national heroine. Source D tells you her first impressions of Scutari Hospital.

Q2 Study Source D. Explain how Florence Nightingale reduced the death rate in Scutari Hospital to 2 per cent.

Drunkenness was very common among the staff nurses, who chiefly were of charwoman type, frequently of bad character, with little education. Nursing, as you understand it now, was unknown. Patients were not nursed, they were attended to, more or less. The work was hard – lockers and tables to scrub every day. We did not scrub the floors. The patients had their beds made once a day, and you thought nothing of changing 14 or 15 poultices two or three times a day. The nurses never used a thermometer, the dressers and clerks took the temperatures.

Source C

An account of nursing in St Bartholomew's Hospital in 1877. It was written in 1902 by a nurse who had been a sister in the hospital in the 1870s.

We now have four miles of beds – and not 18 inches apart. As I went on my night-rounds among the newly wounded that first night, there was not one murmur, the strictest discipline prevailed. These poor fellows bear pain with heroism.

Sometimes, the roof is blown off our quarters, or the windows blown in – and we're flooded and under water for the night. I hope in a few days we shall establish a little cleanliness. …

It appears that in these hospitals the washing of linen and of the men are considered a minor detail. No washing has been performed for the men or the bed – except by ourselves. When we came here, there was neither basin, towel, nor soap in the Wards. The consequences of this are Fever, Cholera, Gangrene, Lice, Bugs, Fleas …

This morning I went into the Purveyor's store. No mops, no plates, no knives and forks, no scissors (for cutting the men's hair which is literally alive) – no basins, no towelling, no Chloride of Lime.
Will you send us
1000 mops
3000 tin plates, 500 dishes
2000 yards of towelling, 200 pairs of scissors
50 quart bottles of disinfecting Chloride of Lime.

Source D

Extracts from letters Florence Nightingale wrote to the British Government after she arrived at Scutari in 1854.

CASE STUDY

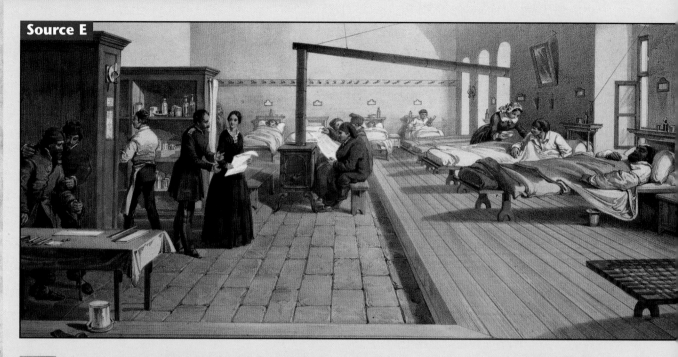
Source E

Study Source E. Is it reliable evidence that Florence Nightingale had carried out her improvements?

A 19th-century painting of Scutari Hospital after Florence Nightingale had carried out her improvements.

Florence Nightingale in Britain

After she returned to Britain in 1856, Nightingale made two major contributions to medicine – establishing nursing as a proper profession, and suggesting ways in which hospitals could be better designed.

Nursing

On her return Nightingale raised £44,000 to set up a nursing school at St Thomas's Hospital. The first students entered in 1860. Her aim was to turn nursing into a respectable profession for women and to produce matrons who would go into hospitals and take control of nursing away from men. For her, nursing was the most important weapon against disease. Nurses could introduce hygiene which would stop infection spreading in hospitals. To do this nurses had to be properly trained. Nursing was not something that any woman could do naturally.

It appears that in these hospitals the washing of linen and of the men are considered a minor detail. No washing has been preformed for the men or the bed- except by ourselves. When we came here, there was neither basin, towel, nor soap in the Wards. The consequences of this are Fever, Cholera, Gangrene, Lice, Bugs, Fleas.

Source F

Nightingale's first letter to Herbert on 25 November 1854.

Miss Nightingale knew that what was needed was radical reform of the whole machinery of hospital and sanitary administration within the army. Besides her nursing she was organising cooking, washing and the distribution of stores while pursuing a running battle with the officials of the Purveyor's Department. Her important contribution was one of organisation – she completely changed the way the hospital was run. She made the ordering of supplies easier. She also organised educational facilities for the wounded soldiers and made sure their wives and children back in Britain were cared for.

Source G

From a recent history book.

In 1859 Nightingale published *Notes on Nursing*. This set down the training that nurses should receive and became the guide for nursing schools for many years. Her ideas had an influence well into the 20th century.

- Like Chadwick she thought sanitation was the key. She believed that proper sanitation, ventilation and the right food would defeat sickness. This meant the training was very practical and ward based.

- She never accepted germ theory and did not allow doctors to give nurses lectures about bacteria. She did not want them becoming 'medical women' with their heads filled with theory. Their job was sanitation.

- She started training women as midwives. The death rate of mothers in maternity wards was very high and the introduction of her methods brought it down.

- By the year 1900 nursing schools had opened around the country, all using Nightingale's ideas.

- Hospitals began to replace mere attendants with properly trained nurses. This led to improved sanitation in hospitals and as a result they became safer places. This meant that the rich were longer worried about going into them and hospitals were able to attract fee paying patients. Hospitals were becoming generally accepted.

The siting and design of hospitals

In 1863 Florence Nightingale published *Notes on Hospitals*. This introduced new ideas about the siting and design of hospitals. When St Thomas's Hospital was demolished she fought for the new hospital to be re-built in the healthy air of the countryside. When it was rebuilt (in London) it had the pavilion ward she had designed. This allowed cross-ventilation because she believed stagnant air bred disease. Countries from all round the world consulted her about plans for new hospitals and many were designed with the needs of sanitation to the forefront.

Q4 Study all the sources. Which is the more accurate description of Nightingale; 'the Lady of the Lamp' or 'an organiser and administrator'? Use the sources to support your answer.

DUTIES OF PROBATIONER

You are required to be sober, honest, punctual, quiet and clean and neat. You are expected to become skilful:

1 In the dressing of blisters, burns, sores, wounds, and in minor dressings.
2 In the application of leeches.
3 In the management of helpless patients, i.e. moving, changing, personal cleanliness of, feeding, and preventing and dressing bed-sores.
4 In bandaging and making bandages.
5 You are required to attend at operations.
6 To understand ventilation, keeping the ward fresh; to observe cleanliness in all utensils.
7 To make observations of the sick: the pulse, appetite, breathing, state of wounds, effect of diet and medicines.

Source H

What student nurses were expected to learn during their training at the Nightingale School of Nursing. This was printed on the back of the application.

CASE STUDY

Mary Seacole

Mary Seacole was another nurse who made her mark in the Crimean War. She was born in Jamaica in 1805. Seacole followed in her mother's footsteps in becoming a doctress. She acted as a midwife and treated the sick using herbal medicine. While she was in Panama cholera broke out and she was the only person there who had any idea of what to do. She ventilated the sick rooms, cleared away filth and vermin and isolated the patients from each other. She even carried out surgery dealing with gunshot wounds. By the 1850s she had gathered an enormous amount of medical knowledge and experience.

In 1854 Seacole arrived in Britain and volunteered her services to the army in the Crimea. She waited weeks without even being interviewed so she decided to go to the Crimea at her own expense. When she arrived she set up her 'British Hotel'. Here Seacole supplied soldiers with clean and nourishing food and drink. She dealt with jaundice, diarrhoea, dysentery and frostbite and was often seen going into the thick of battle with her medicine bag, where she treated all kinds of wounds. She quickly won the love and respect of the soldiers.

When the war ended in 1856 Seacole was left with large amounts of stock which she could not sell. She returned to Britain and was made bankrupt. *The Times* and other newspapers took up her cause and published letters from ex-soldiers telling how they owed their lives to her. A huge four-day benefit concert was held to raise money for her. Tens of thousands of people attended but the company organising the event went bankrupt and Seacole ended up with just £233. In 1857, however, she published her memoirs and when she died in 1881 she was quite well off. Unfortunately, apart from her work as a masseuse to members of the royal family, no more use was made of her great medical experience and knowledge.

How different were the skills and experience which Mary Seacole and Florence Nightingale brought to the suffering army. At the base hospitals in Scutari, Florence's main role was organising. Regulations and tradition prevented nurses from performing any but the most basic duties. They were engaged in undoing bandages, washing wounds before inspection by the medical officer, spoon-feeding patients and comforting the terminally ill. They were rarely seen outside the wards. Mary threw herself into the work of relieving the suffering among the troops. There were times when she refused to wait for the cease-fire but carefully picked her way through the mutilated bodies of men hit by shot and shell, seeking out the wounded and dying, whether enemy or ally.

Source I

From a book about Mary Seacole published in 1984.

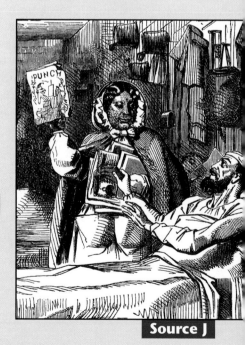

Source J

Mary Seacole as drawn in 'Punch' magazine, May 1857.

EXAM PRACTICE QUESTIONS

(a) How similar was the work of Florence Nightingale and Mary Seacole in the Crimea?

(b) Florence Nightingale believed in the miasma theory. Explain how this influenced her work and ideas about hospitals.

(c) Who made the more important contribution to the development of medicine, Florence Nightingale or Mary Seacole?

The 18th to 20th Centuries

Factors

- The development of industry led to new machines, materials and chemicals being developed e.g. better glass for microscopes, drugs like Salverson 606, and allowed penicillin to be mass produced

- The needs of French industry gave Pasteur opportunities to carry out research

- National rivalry made Pasteur and Koch compete against each other

- Chance helped Pasteur to discover how vaccination works and Fleming to discover penicillin

- Teamwork helped Pasteur and Koch – in modern science no one could be an expert in every field, people needed to share their expertise

- War helped and hindered the development of penicillin and speeded up the development of plastic surgery

- Diseases such as cholera forced governments to act over public health

- The working classes getting the vote made governments do more about public health

- Governments became more involved e.g. taking responsibility for public health, setting up the NHS

- The gathering of statistics about people's health by people like Booth and Rowntree led to public health reforms

- Brilliant individuals like Pasteur, Fleming and Simpson

Ideas about disease

- At the beginning of the 19th century people believed disease was spread by miasma (bad air)

- Others believed in spontaneous generation

- Pasteur proved the germ theory

Other points

- Many of the developments of this period faced strong opposition: vaccination, anaesthetics, antiseptics, germ theory and public health reform were all opposed.

- Modern medicine has brought its own problems

- There are still many medical problems to be overcome

Today's problems

New treatments

Penicillin kills a wide range of germs but not all. Other antibiotics have been developed e.g. for tuberculosis. Many different kinds of living organisms have been used to produce them e.g cephalosporins were developed from a mould found in sea water near a sewer. Vaccines have been developed against measles, mumps, typhoid, German measles, whooping cough and polio.

Gene therapy is an exciting development – many illnesses are caused by a defect in a single gene and can be treated by introducing into the body undamaged copies of the gene. We all have about 10,000 genes. The Human Gene Project is mapping them all – we will then be able to identify the defect causing every inherited disorder, and correct it.

And there are other problems

Some diseases such as malaria have gradually become resistant to drugs. They have the ability to adapt themselves – some are already resistant to penicillin. Antibiotics are also expensive. In Britain the NHS will not prescribe some drugs because of the expense and many people in developing countries are deprived of these drugs because of the cost.

But some drugs have side effects

Cortisone, a drug developed for rheumatoid arthritis, has enabled people to walk again but it has also caused heart disease and stomach ulcers. The biggest disaster was Thalidomide, a drug introduced in the late 1950s to help people sleep. By 1961 it was clear that if it was taken by women during pregnancy it caused serious damage to foetuses in the womb. Over 10,000 babies were born whose arms and legs had not developed. The drug was withdrawn and laws were passed making drug companies test new drugs more vigorously.

Old killer, new killers

First the good news

In the developed world life expectation has increased dramatically. It went up in Britain from 45 to 75 during the 20th century. The main reason for this was the decline in the number of people dying from infectious diseases. In the 19th century the biggest cause of death was infectious disease – one death in every three. Infectious disease now accounts for 0.5 per cent of all deaths. Improvements in sanitation, hygiene, living conditions and nutrition have been the most important factors in reducing the number of deaths from diseases such as tuberculosis, cholera and dysentery, while vaccination has almost totally eliminated polio, measles, mumps, whooping cough, tetanus and German measles.

Now the bad news

However, new killer diseases have replaced the old ones. Some of the major new killers are brought about by our lifestyle. Through most of the 20th century, there was an increase in the number of people smoking. It is the main cause of lung cancer and other forms of lung disease.

It has been estimated that by 2025 smoking will kill ten million people – half of all regular smokers will be killed by the habit. In the USA one thousand people a day die from smoking-related diseases. Governments fail to take tougher action against smoking because of the vast amount of taxes they collect from cigarettes. Should smoking be made illegal?

Other major killers are cancer and heart disease. What is so worrying about the figures in Source A is that we could do much to prevent them. Heart disease is brought about by cholesterol fatty deposits in the arteries and could be reduced by eating less saturated fat, stopping smoking and taking more exercise.

It gets worse

New infections have also appeared such as legionnaire's disease and AIDS. The latter appeared in the 1970s in Africa. It affects the body's immune system by reducing its defences against attack so patients often die from infections such as tuberculosis or tumours. It is caused by HIV, a virus which is transmitted by sexual contact, infected blood, or across the placenta from an infected mother to unborn child.

No vaccine or cure has yet been developed. By 1996 over 30 million people had HIV, many of them children and 19 million of them in Africa. Eight million people had, by then, died of AIDS.

	1911	1992
deaths from cancer	37,700 (7% of all deaths)	146,000 (26% of all deaths)
heart disease	83,000 (16% of all deaths)	255,000 (46% of all deaths)

Source A

Deaths from all forms of cancer and from heart disease in Britain.

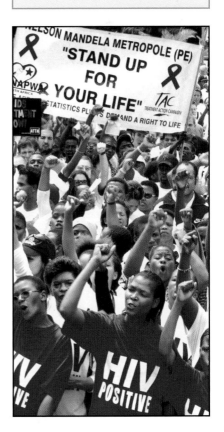

Source B

AIDS activists protesting in South Africa in February 2003. They were worried that the government appeared to be ignoring the AIDS pandemic that was ravaging the country.

The developing world

Let's start with a bit of good news

The World Health Organisation has eradicated smallpox worldwide by a programme of vaccination. Other programmes are underway to eradicate measles, whooping cough and polio but in parts of Africa and in India (where 22 million children are born each year) only about half the children are vaccinated.

And now the bad news

While we make ourselves ill by smoking, overeating, overdrinking and taking little exercise people in the developing world die through no fault of their own. See Source C.

In the developing world two million children die each year from measles and three million from diarrhoeal diseases. Diphtheria, polio, dysentery and tuberculosis are still killers. More and more people are arguing that instead of trying to introduce expensive western drugs and high-tech medicine, far more could be done by more basic measures – a piped supply of clean water, simple education of mothers about health care, childhood immunisation. Just adding salt and sugar to water to prevent dehydration, from which three million children die a year, would save many lives. Much more needs to be done. Some argue that the world's resources need to be shared much more equally, but will people in the developed world ever agree to this?

With little sign of birth rates in the developing world falling, some doctors are beginning to ask some very difficult questions. Take the example of the oral rehydration of children suffering from severe diarrhoea. An individual doctor may be duty bound, they say, to rehydrate a child in their care, but some doctors argue that a large scheme to do this over a wide area should not be set up because it will simply increase the years of misery for many people who will eventually die of starvation. What is the point of denying infants a quick death when all they face as adults is a lingering and more painful death? Do you agree?

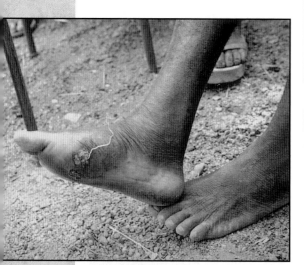

Source D

The guinea worm is a parasite that grows beneath the skin, sometimes to a length of 60 centimetres. It causes pain and disability to some ten million people in Africa and Asia. Clean drinking water would defeat it.

Source C

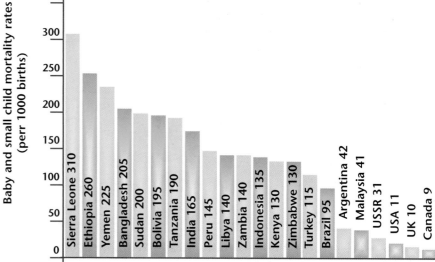

Baby and small child mortality rates (perr 1000 births)

Sierra Leone 310, Ethiopia 260, Yemen 225, Bangladesh 205, Sudan 200, Bolivia 195, Tanzania 190, India 165, Peru 145, Libya 140, Zambia 140, Indonesia 135, Kenya 130, Zimbabwe 130, Turkey 115, Brazil 95, Argentina 42, Malaysia 41, USSR 31, USA 11, UK 10, Canada 9

Infant mortality in different countries in 1960.

The NHS in crisis

The National Health Service has provided free health care in Britain for people who otherwise would not be able to afford it.

But the NHS is in desperate trouble. Waiting lists for operations are getting longer and doctors and nurses are overworked. Many hospitals need modernising and are struggling to cope with the demands on their services.

The main problem is money. When it was set up the NHS was expected to cost £170 million a year. By 1960 it was costing £726 million a year, by 1990 £3500 million. Modern medicine and drugs are very expensive. The number of elderly people is fast increasing. They use the NHS much more than young people. Also, the birth rate has been dropping, which means there are fewer people in work to pay for the NHS. Should taxes be increased to pay for a better NHS or should more people pay for their own medical treatment?

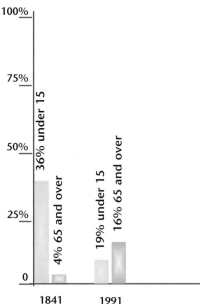

Source E

The graph shows that the proportion of Britain's population that is elderly is growing fast.

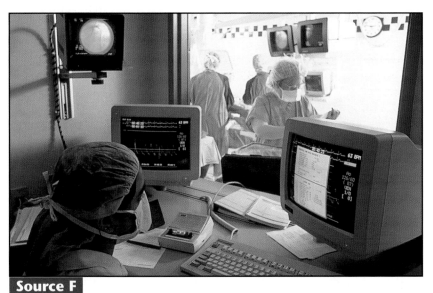

Source F

Unblocking a coronary artery – an example of today's expensive treatment. Using X-ray images a small balloon on the end of a fine tube is threaded through a vein and into the blocked artery. The balloon is pumped up, clearing the artery. The operation is monitored in the control room.

There are many other issues!

Should we be keeping people alive for as long as possible? What is the point of doing this when it means old people will have extra years suffering from diseases such as Alzheimer's and Parkinson's? Should those living in pain and disability be allowed to choose voluntary euthanasia?

Through genetic screening we can now diagnose inherited disorders before birth. Should all foetuses be screened? Should pregnancies be terminated when disorders are found?

You can see that, despite all the developments in medicine over thousands of years, we are still faced with many problems!